# CONVERSATION FAILURE
## CASE STUDIES IN
## DOCTOR-PATIENT COMMUNICATION

Frederic W. Platt, M.D.

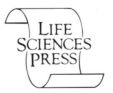

Life Sciences Press
Tacoma, WA

Life Sciences Press, P.O. Box 1174, Tacoma, WA 98401

Made in the United States of America

Library of Congress Cataloging-in-Publication Data


Platt, Frederic W.
    Conversation failure - case studies in doctor-patient
communication / Frederic W. Platt
        p.   cm.
    Includes bibliographical references.
    ISBN 0-943685-126-8 : $16.95
    1. Physician and patient--Case studies.  2. Medical history
taking--Case studies.  I. Title.
R727.3.P495 1992
610.69'6--dc20                                    92-15049
                                                      CIP


ISBN 0-943685-16-8


Cover art by: Lund-Katke Group, San Clemente, CA

# TABLE OF CONTENTS

This book is dedicated to the memory of my uncle,
Joe Linn,
a man who didn't like doctors.

# ACKNOWLEDGEMENTS

My thanks go to all my medical teachers and patients who have, gradually, over many years, led me to understand better what happens when doctors and patients converse.

I thank Greg Carroll, Vaughn Keller, and Pamela Rowland-Morin of the Miles Pharmaceuticals Program on Doctor-Patient Communication for their encouragement and their wonderful ideas.

I have been blessed with a colleague in the practice of medicine who has shared most of my medical adventures, joined with me in sorting out diagnoses and conversational pitfalls, and always been a support and an inspiration. I give bushels of thanks to Dr. A. Lee Anneberg, who has been my constant ally and support in the practice of medicine.

Dr. Geoffrey Gordon of the University of Oregon and the Portland V.A. Hospital has been a great help with this written work. He is very conscious of the communication struggle of physician and patient and of their desire for a better outcome. Many of his suggestions have blended into my discussions, leaving him precious little credit for the amount of help he gave. I thank him.

And thank you to my publisher Alexander G. Schauss and assistant, Laura Babin for their interest and help in publishing *Conversation Failure*.

Most of all, I want to thank my wife, Constance Platt. Her awareness of the human issues of medicine, her gentle prompting, and her guidance over thirty years have helped me to be a better person and a better doctor. And her thoughtful editing of this work has made it more readable and hopefully more fun for others.

Several of the cases in this book have been published elsewhere. I thank the publishers for permission to reprint them here. *PATIENT CARE* for "Acute Myelocytic Leukemia," "I AN ALK I OU I EEH," "How Can I Trust You?" and "Please Step This Way"; Miles Pharmaceutical Co. *COMMENT* for "Just a Cold" and "A Rash is A Rash"; Little, Brown for "Terrible Sore Throat", from *Case Studies in Emergency Medicine*, Second Edition, 1991; and the Saint Joseph Hospital *PRIMARY CARE BULLETIN* for "Big Talker," "How Smart Are You," and "No Traditional Doctor."

Frederic W. Platt, M.D.
1992

# FOREWORD

We have been teaching medical students interviewing techniques for decades. We teach such courses in the first two years of medical school and buttress them with good textbooks, of which there are many. However, few students read these textbooks. In fact, students often put low priority on interview courses. They enjoy the contact with patients but know that their grades come from other courses that therefore must be more important.

When students begin their clinical rotations they quickly learn from interns and residents what is really important. The techniques they then acquire include very directive, yes-no questions and limited inquiry about the patient's experience or life setting of illness. If they previously credited devices such as open-ended questions, eliciting the patient's concerns and ideas, or empathy, they now discard such devices as impractical due to time pressures.

As interns and residents, trainees may feel overwhelmed by the amount of knowledge and skills to master to care for seriously ill patients. Interviewing skills translate into an ever-expanding list of questions to ask, a huge review of systems. House officers often view other aspects of the interview as a matter of personal style and as such become defensive about criticism or suggestions. Their teachers rarely observe them talking with patients except during brief bedside round contacts and occasional clinical competency examinations.

Finally, as practicing physicians, we begin to recognize that problems occur in our interactions with patients and that we lack techniques or procedures to handle these problems. Practicing physicians have seldom read the current literature on medical interviewing, have not attended workshops in the field, and have forgotten those introductory textbooks. We have accumulated a wealth of examples of doctor-patient conversation failure and we tend to blame the patient most of the time for such failures. We might learn from these failures but we have no forum in which to share them.

In this book, Dr. Fred Platt draws on decades of dialogues with patients and colleagues to bring us a useful and entertaining collection of doctor-patient conversation mishaps. These are arranged as independent vignettes that can be read much like a newspaper's daily bridge column. These dialogues will ring true for doctors and patients alike. After reading each vignette, I suggest that you think about WHAT WENT WRONG in the conversation and WHY, and what you might have said or done differently. Then read the author's discussion of the possible causes and solutions.

I think you will find Fred Platt's writing style to be friendly and open. He is forgiving and respectful of patients and doctors, including himself. This entertaining and instructive book provides a painless approach to understanding doctor-patient communication. It is a useful addition to the current literature and to textbooks on medical interviewing.

Geoffrey H. Gordon, M.D.
Staff Physician, Portland Veteran's Hospital Medical Center
Associate Professor of Medicine and Psychiatry
University of Oregon

# PREFACE

Both physicians and patients tell of frequent communication mishaps; they differ largely in whom they blame, each crediting the other for the problem.[1,2,3] I believe that communication problems arise frequently and that whatever the cause, it is our task as physicians to address them.[4] A reasonable approach for a doctor dealing with conversation failure is to follow standard medical procedure: determine what is going wrong, then devise a treatment for it.

The title of this book is CONVERSATION FAILURE. But the meat of the book is conversation repair.

This book contains 71 clinical vignettes and dialogues, transcribed after real patient encounters. I have simplified the dialogues for better focus, removing hesitations and garbled transmissions, even though I realize that some linguistic precision may be lost. I have changed names, shortened dialogues, and occasionally combined two conversations into one. Nonetheless, each example has the validity of having happened at least once. If the reader recognizes the interaction from his or her own practice, she can be sure that the problem has arisen at least twice.

As you read these dialogues, pause at the end of each case presentation and ask yourself, what is going wrong? Then ask, what might I do at this point to clarify the problem and to remedy it? After formulating your own solution, read the discussion.

I have had help with these discussions. I have been assisted by other clinicians, by the patients themselves, and by scientists who study clinical interactions and communication process. And the solutions I suggest to these clinical puzzles are not the only possible ones. Even though I make definite recommendations, I realize that there are other reasonable ways to approach the specific conversational problem and perhaps other reasonable diagnoses of just what that problem is. Conversational techniques are often dependent on the personal styles of the people involved. If a procedure or technique that I describe seems uncomfortable to the reader, it may be only because it is new to him and will become more comfortable with use. Or it may be that the specific technique is not really for him or her. It is best to view these dialogues as difficult challenges just like in-person interviews, and to keep an open mind and an experimental attitude toward the process.

These cases are not ordered in any logical sequence. They provide the same random collection of interview challenges as our daily patients. We don't see all our incoherent patients on Monday and all our angry ones on Tuesday.

Although this book makes no pretense of adequately summarizing the extensive literature about doctor-patient communication, I have inserted some favorite references for the reader who wishes further clarification. To begin, I have listed some of my favorite textbooks dealing with medical communication.[A-Q]

I am concerned that the reader may find my discussions too caustic, blaming the doctor in the dialogue. In fact, I think that we all have these same problems and that blame is the last thing we need. We all carry around too many critical messages and I hope that we will come to feel less guilty for our misses and our slips. No one can bat 1.000, especially in this difficult arena, but it is fair to try to improve our averages and we can do that with increased awareness of conversational pitfalls and armed with better communication techniques.

Are all interactional problems between doctor and patient amenable to this sort of analysis? Surely not. Not all problem patients represent mere conversational failures. Personality disorders, psychoses, and other psychiatric illnesses make for difficult communication. However, even with such severe psychopathology, many of the devices apply.

Finally, I would say that I view interview process as a subject of technical scrutiny and the skills involved as a learnable technology. Interview technique does not come naturally to most of us. It is a collection of learned skills, enjoyable to practice and beneficial to patients, who are all worthy of our best efforts at hearing and learning from them.

I hope that my insights are useful to my readers. If so, they will have more fun with the practice of medicine and be more helpful to their patients.

# I DON'T LIKE DOCTORS

Dr. Xylom: Hello, you must be Mr. Linn. I'm Dr. Xylom.

L: I'm glad to meet you Doctor.

X: Let's start by having you tell me a little about yourself.

L: Well, first you have to know that I don't like doctors.

X: Uh huh?

L: I think they are all high priced mechanics. The only doctor I like at all is my nephew and he's in Denver.

X: And where do you live?

L: I've lived in Wilmette the last 20 years.

X: Yes? What do you do?

L: I'm retired. I used to own a men's hotel. Now I don't do anything but sit around and maybe play a little poker or pinochle every so often.

X: And what sort of troubles are you having?

L: Most of my troubles are my doctors. They all want to do tests and procedures and send their bills. That's about all they care about.

X: No medical troubles?

L: Sure. I've got emphysema and I had heart disease. They fixed that with an angioplasty but I still get pain if I walk upstairs without a nitro. And I have to use oxygen all the time. I puff terribly and can't move without it. Mostly I'm sick all the time from all the pills you guys push on me.

X: Well, let's see if I can list all your medicines. Tell me what you are taking.


Dr. X. says that this is his least favorite sort of patient. He says that he feels one down from the start, trying to deal with a patient who has announced his dislike and distrust of doctors.

What do you think? What would you advise Dr. X. to do?

## DISCUSSION

Dr. Xylom says that he finds this sort of patient immensely frustrating. I can imagine that it feels painful. But I wonder if Dr. Xylom isn't taking too much pain onto himself. After all, this patient hasn't ever met Dr. Xylom before. His comments describe himself, his own lack of trust in doctors, perhaps his past experiences.

So what could one do with this declaration? The doctor in this conversation chose to disregard his patient's every remark about doctors. He thought them either a joke or evidence of hostility, and that the best strategy with either would be to bypass the remark, disregard it.

We should never do that. We must take our patients seriously, even their jokes. They are telling us something important. We should never disregard them or their comments.

Besides, this sort of remark is a gift. We can be grateful to this patient who has opened himself to us this way. We don't have to struggle to detect latent hostility when he fails, later, to comply with our instructions. We can take this gift now, explore it, defuse it, and use it to build a therapeutic relationship.

Dr. X: You don't like doctors?

L: Well, some of them are OK. But I think most of my troubles come from the medicines. And I have yet to meet a doctor who listens to me.

X: So it seems that doctors seldom really listen to you. And you are concerned that your troubles may come partly from your medicines.

L: That's it, Doctor.

X: Is there more? More bad experiences with doctors?

L: Oh, yeah. I've had several I wouldn't take a dog to, even a dog I didn't like. A couple of cardiologists who were convinced they were God's gift to the human race.

X: So sometimes doctors have been offensive in their self-importance?

L: Yeah, well, you know I don't think any doctor has ever asked me how I felt about doctors before.

X: They probably never listened to you saying you didn't like doctors.

L: They didn't have time.

How powerful the alliance is already! What an opportunity this sort of remark from the patient is! We must stay alert for these remarks.

# *ASLEEP*

Dr. Terry:  Hello, I'm Dr. Terry.  Are you Mr. Ymage?

Y:  Uh, uh — yeah. (Sleeping in bed in a darkened room, he barely opens one eye.)

T:  I need to talk with you. I'd like you to tell me what sort of trouble you've been having.

Y:  Uh, uh.

T:  Why did you come here?

Y:  It hurt. It's better now.

T:  Tell me more about this hurting, can you?

Y:  Yeah, over here. (points to his flank in a vague way)

T:  Go on.

Y:  Woke me up. Terrible.

[silence — finally, after one minute pause]

T:  Can you tell me more?

Y:  (clearly sleeping)

## DISCUSSION

This case was first published in 1979.[5] I noted at that time that the case seemed trivial but exemplified a common and important problem. The interviewer was having trouble with a sleepy patient who had recently been given a narcotic and was resting in a darkened room. It seemed that the doctor had not formulated any hypothesis about his patient's nonresponsiveness since he took no steps to improve the situation. Turning the lights on or sitting the patient up might have helped. This interviewer was an excellent doctor; his inability to deal with a trivial difficulty surprised me.

This was the first time I began to realize that physicians could benefit by trying to diagnose and treat problem interviews, that such an effort could serve as a unifying approach for interview problems. Prior to this case I believed that most problem interviews were the doctor's fault. I was impressed that the doctor often introduced difficulties by being untherapeutic, by high-pressure interviewing techniques, by failing to insist on primary data, and by not being thorough enough. This case and others like it led me to realize that the doctor would be better armed if he or she simply spent a little time noting that the interview was not going well and considering why that might be.

I thought that it would be reasonable to have a differential diagnosis of why interviews go wrong and suggested the following list:

> The patient is
>> confused
>> asleep or sleepy
>> very sick, perhaps urgently so
>> a theorist
>> tangential
>> circumstantial
>> telling a saga of medical care
>> angry
>> depressed
>> denying symptoms or their significance
>> concerned with an urgent need
>> psychotic
>> deaf, mute, aphasic, or a non-English speaker
>> busy, e.g. on a bed pan
>> missing critical items of communication (glasses, teeth, hearing aid)
>
> There are
>> distractions in the room, e.g. noisy TV set
>> relatives or friends adding to story or confusion
>> relatives or friends who perceive an urgent need

That list is still reasonable. We might update it by adding

> Other system problems:
>> doctor-doctor communication
>> hospital or insurance program
>> ambulance system (kidnappings, information loss)
>
> Doctor-generated communication difficulties:
>> non-therapeutic doctor
>> high pressure interview, leaving patient little room to tell his story
>> incomplete history taking
>> failure to demand primary data

Timothy Quill has also attempted to devise a taxonomy of the difficulties a physician faces in communicating with patients.[6] One might consider amalgamating the two lists of communication problems. But I don't believe that either or both of us have accounted for all doctor-patient interview mishaps. Better than holding a list in mind is probably just the awareness that things do go wrong and that we can think our way out of the difficulty if we spend some time doing just that, thinking about it.

Dr. Terry might have been asleep at the switch with this sleepy patient, but he was razor sharp at other times. I observed him one morning, meeting Ms. Stern on rounds.

T: Good morning, Ms. Stern, how are you today?

S: Awful, Doctor. They haven't brought me my morning coffee yet. I don't talk to anyone until I've had my morning coffee.

T: Well, can you talk with me?

S: Nope. I'm just a bear until I have my coffee.

Then Dr. Terry did something brilliant. He said "OK," and he left the room, returning in two minutes with a steaming cup of coffee for her. That act became a model to me of how one human can respond to another, as fine doctors do.

# IS THIS WHY I WENT TO MEDICAL SCHOOL?

Dr. P: Hello, you must be Ms. Grape. I'm Dr. Platt. I'm an internist, an internal medicine doctor, and your regular physician here at The Rehab Center asked me to visit with you, to examine you, and to assist in your care. This is Dr. Smith, a student doctor who is working with me. He will just listen in to our conversation if that is OK with you.

Ms. Grape: Humph. (She doesn't face the doctor; sits with her head facing away from him even though he is facing her. Her language is terse and flat in affect. She sounds angry or distrustful.)

Dr. P: Well, if you are comfortable in the chair there, we can begin. Is this OK with you?

Ms. G: Humph.

Dr. P: All right, let's begin by finding out a little bit about you. Where are you from?

[Long Pause]

Ms. G: Texas... But I moved up here 'cause my brother and my sister are up here.

Dr. P: OK, and what do you do?

[Pause]

Ms. G: You mean work?

Dr. P: Yeah.

Ms. G: Well I ain't done no work for a while. Before I was a nurse's aide. I worked in a nursing home. I had to get the bodies cleaned up when they died. And I did housekeeping and custodian.

Dr. P: And are you married?

[Pause]

Ms. G: Single.

Dr. P: I see. And what happened that got you into the hospital?

[Pause]

Ms. G: (Still turned half away from the doctor as she has been throughout the interview) I was beat up and left out in the field and I froze my feet.

[Pause]

Dr. P: Oh my, that must have been terrible. How are you feeling now?

Ms. G: My feet hurt. They hurt in the toes and the tops and the ankles. And I got headaches all the time and I can't concentrate and they're going to do a MRI to see if my brain was damaged.

Dr. P: When did that happen to you?

Ms. G: What? The rape and beating? That wasn't the first time.

Dr. P: You had been beaten before? Raped?

[Pause]

Ms. G: Well raped anyway. Never froze before.

Dr. P: That all sounds painful. How did it happen?

[Pause]

Ms. G: Do I have to talk about it?

Dr. P: Is it hard? Perhaps you can tell me the main points.

Ms. G: I told them already.

Dr. P: OK, perhaps we can get back to it if we have to. How are you feeling now? Mostly sad? Mostly angry?

Ms. G: Just hurt, that's all. My feet hurts.

Dr. P: All right. What other troubles are you having?

Ms. G: That's all. I don't think straight.

Dr. P: In what way?

[Pause]

Ms. G: I don't remember everything all the time.

Dr. P: Hmm. I wonder. Are you angry now? Are you angry with me?

[Pause]

Ms. G: (sounds angry) What would I be angry with you for? I never saw you before.

Dr. P: Yes, that's right. I had the feeling that perhaps you were angry, Ms. Grape.

Ms. G: No.

Dr. P: OK, tell me a little more about your health. Smoke?

Ms. G: No. Not ever.

Dr. P: Drink? Alcohol?

Ms. G: Sure, I drink. Not much though.

Dr. P: How much would you guess you might drink in an average week?

Ms. G: I can't even guess at that.

Dr. P: Can you tell me what you drink? Beer? Wine? Vodka?

Ms. G:  I don't know.  It all depends.

Dr. P:  OK, what I've heard then is that you were beaten, raped, and left out all night, freezing your feet. Now your feet and ankles hurt a lot. You've been raped before. You don't smoke but you do drink some, but you're not sure how much. Is that right?

Ms. G:  Yeah.

(She still is facing away from the doctor, still nearly monosyllabic, still sounds angry and distrusting.)

Dr. P:  When was this last beating? The time your feet were injured.

Ms. G:  February 26th.

Dr. P:  And now, how long have you been here at The Rehab Center?

Ms. G:  I came in last Thursday.

Dr. P:  So, almost a week. And in the past, other than the times you've told me about, have you been in hospital or had operations?

Ms. G:  Just for my kids.  And I had two hysterectomies.  And my tonsils and my appendix.

Dr. P:  You have kids?

Ms. G:  Yeah. Five. The oldest boy's run off. The others is with my sister and with my mother.

Dr. P:  And do you take any medicines or drugs?

Ms. G:  Just Tylenol.  They give me stuff here in the hospital but they stopped it all and now I ain't vomiting so much.

Dr. P:  You were vomiting? When was that?

Ms. G:  Until yesterday. Not today.

Dr. P:  Sounds like stopping the medicines was maybe a good idea. What other troubles are you having?

Ms. G:  Just my feet hurt.


# DISCUSSION

This conversation was a surprise to me. Feeling confident in my ability to interview patients, I had brought a medical student along with me. The student was finishing his second year and had joined me for a brief tune-up of examination skills prior to his clinical years. I thought it reasonable for him to observe a master at work. As Geoff Gordon puts it, I was "ready to do the biopsychosocial cosmic interview." Much to my surprise, this patient offered a degree of difficulty that nearly finished me off. What a joke, I thought, realizing that she might, at any moment, refuse to cooperate at all. Perhaps this student will be fortunate enough to see that no matter how practiced the doctor, he can fail. Everyone can have a bad day and everyone can meet his or her match.

Once it was clear that something was going wrong, I was sure that my patient was angry with me. I thought that she was probably angry with others or with life and that the anger was overflowing onto me. But that interpretation seemed to go nowhere with her. It was hard for me to let loose of that interpretation. Giving up an erroneous diagnosis was harder for me than formulating one, especially since I had no better one to replace it with. Still, I should know that when I offer an interpretation and it fails to yield a positive response from my patient, I am usually wrong.

The other diagnosis I considered, an incomplete one, was that my patient was very fragile. Accordingly, I tried to treat her as gently as I could, which allowed us to progress, tentatively, through the interview. Only during the physical examination did I get a better understanding of the patient's affect. I noted that she found it hard to let me uncover her for the examination. She kept covering up parts I had uncovered. "Aha!" I thought. "She is frightened."

Why should it be so difficult for me to recognize fear in a woman who is in a strange city, in a strange environment, surrounded by powerful people she doesn't know or trust after having had the terrible experience of beating, rape, and abandonment? And her attacker was, of course, another man. Surely fear is every bit as common as anger. I wonder why it was so hard for me to recognize it? Fear is usually contagious and I surely felt uncomfortable during the interview, but I was unable to diagnose my own discomfort as fear. Once I did realize that she was frightened, I could say to her, "You have had a terrible experience and I can imagine that all of this is still fearful to you. It must be very frightening."

That did the trick. She actually looked at me and nodded yes. And, as in so many of these miraculous empathetic connections, her cooperation increased and she suddenly seemed to gain a great deal of trust. She later even thanked me for coming to see her.

So, in the end, the student did witness a little bit of magic. And I felt more humble. Had the presence of an audience been a distraction to me? I didn't think so, since I had lost all sense of the student's presence midway into the interview. I think my failure to understand the patient came from my lack of flexibility and my message to myself is "Keep awake. If one explanation fails to fit, consider others. And while thinking, act gently."

During the interview, feeling strained and unable to master the problem, I wondered, was this why I went to medical school? Surely I hadn't done all that work, and the work of residency, and the work since, to be obliged to suffer this way at the hands of this patient? Of course that is a self-centered way to think of the situation. The patient is the one who is suffering, not I. If I feel victimized by the process, I am creating that role myself. And it is my job to figure out the problem and resolve it, not to feel myself a victim. Yet the pain of the process is real and we all feel it. Sometimes we hear doctors claiming that they don't like to care for certain patients. More often we blame the patients and give them titles such as 'The Hateful Patient,' all ways to escape from the pain of difficult processes, but none of them solutions. And miraculously, once a solution is found, we feel as I did that yes, indeed, this was exactly why I became a physician, this *was* why I went to medical school.

# FUNNY YOU SHOULD ASK THAT

Dr. P: Mrs. Raven, I am still puzzled. You've got these painful red lumps on the backs of your calves and I haven't got a good idea what is causing them or what to do with them. We did a lot of blood tests and a chest X-ray because I think these are what we call Erythema Nodosum placques, but nothing was abnormal. And I have to admit that that sort of skin lesion usually appears on the front of the calves, not the backs. I wonder if we ought to send you to a dermatologist for a biopsy.

Mrs. R: Whatever you think, doctor.

P: Well, I have an idea. Let me see if Dr. Anneberg is free. He's my partner, you know. Sometimes he has good ideas that I haven't thought of.

[He goes out and shortly returns with Dr. Anneberg in tow.]

P: Lee, let me introduce you to Mrs. Raven. Mrs. R, this is my partner, Dr. Anneberg. Lee, I've been puzzled by her skin lesions. She has these red placques on the backs of her legs. I've never seen E. Nodosum there before.

A: Hmm. What do you rub the backs of your legs on?

R: It's funny you should ask that, doctor.

A: Yes?

R: Well, you know I live up at the shrine on Lookout Mountain. I feed the chickens each day and I have to carry two buckets of feed down about 100 steps on the hillside. I get frightened of the height and usually I can keep from being too scared if I scrape my legs along the steps just behind me. Do you think that is causing the red marks?

How can we avoid such a surprise?

## DISCUSSION

More ominous words are never spoken. For Dr. P., seeking an answer but not expecting it to tumble out so quickly or so easily, the handwriting was on the wall the moment his patient said, "Funny you should ask that."

How often, when one is puzzled about a diagnosis, does clarity come with the answer to a question like, what do you do? It is valuable, especially when you're stumped, to know more about the patient's physical activity, job situation, or home conditions. I've learned amazing facts about work conditions that I would never have imagined just by asking to be told how one goes about the tasks named. Do you know that the job of tying flies might involve pressing a pedal on a machine 10,000 times a day? I didn't, until told. How often a pain is explained by a new athletic activity, a change in shoes, a new golf swing.

Other good questions of this sort include: "What new things have happened to you lately?", "Are you doing anything new?", "Are there any new stresses in your life?", "Any new hobbies?"

Many physicians work in isolation, sharing little of their puzzlements and their fears with another colleague. If you can find a colleague to share with, your emotional and intellectual load will be lightened immediately. These two doctors share a patient or two every day and get great pleasure out of the collaboration. Sometimes there is nothing to say but "I can see how puzzling a problem this is. I'm puzzled too. I think you've done the appropriate tests (or therapy). Let me know if anything comes clear over the next week." Other times a second head is better than the first. This case was clarified immediately with the right question by the second doctor.

# WEEKEND ROUNDS

Dr. Thane: Mr. Salmon? I'm Dr. Thane. I'm making rounds for Dr. Goldberg this weekend. How are you doing?

Mr. S: Not bad, except for the pain.

Dr. T: Tell me about it.

Mr. S: Well, it's the same thing. I have pain here, in the pit of my stomach, and nobody seems to be able to figure it out. In fact, it is getting worse.

Dr. T: I see. You said worse. Worse in what way?

Mr. S: Well mostly it's there more of the time. At first it never woke me up at night. Now it's likely to be there any time. I haven't slept through for weeks.

Dr. T: Does it go anywhere else?

Mr. S: Not really. It sits right here. Sometimes I can't exactly place the pain. After it's been there for an hour or so, sometimes it seems to involve my entire body, front and back.

Dr. T: What do you do when the pain is there?

Mr. S: I've tried antacids, Mylanta and Rolaids and all those. For a while Dr. Anneberg had me taking Tagamet. I even tried those nitro pills that you put under your tongue.

Nothing helped. Not a bit. I went to Dr. Anneberg and he put me into the hospital. He did X-rays and he had Butterworth look down into my stomach with his gastroscope. Anneberg even had me walking a treadmill. That was a month ago but I still got that damn belly pain.

Dr. T: Hmm. And what do you do physically when you get the pain? Lie down? Walk around?

Mr. S: It doesn't seem to matter, but mostly I just lie there.

Dr. T: Huh. And have you found anything that you avoid doing? Anything that the pain prevents?

Mr. S: Well, I sure have looked. But I haven't figured out what brings on the pain and neither have the doctors. They seem as baffled as I am. Dr. Goldberg says he doesn't have a clue.

I don't know if I ought to go somewhere else or what.

Dr. T: Well, I wouldn't worry about it. I'm sure that Dr. Goldberg and Dr. Anneberg will figure it out. They will probably have to do a few more tests.

Mr. S: (suddenly clearly irate) What tests? What tests? I told you, they've done everything they can think of. They can't find out.

Dr. T: Ah, well, I'm going to have to go now. Is there anything else you would like from us?

Mr. S: I would like to know why I have this pain.

Dr. T: Uh huh. Well, I will see you tomorrow. Goodbye.

Mr. S: Goodbye.

## DISCUSSION

In this brief interview, the physicians present all agreed with Dr. Thane that things seemed to be going well until a very specific point when the patient became angry. Dr. Thane was surprised since the problem seemed to arise just when she had done something therapeutic, attempted to reassure him. She even felt a little betrayed by his response.

When asked about the diagnosis and the therapy for this problem, the doctors wondered if Dr. Thane had attempted too much. She could have asked less about his pain and simply fobbed the problem off on his regular doctors. One physician wondered if the pain was perhaps psychogenic and the patient too invested in its physical reality to accept any other explanation. That observer wondered if the patient wasn't fighting to defend his view of the pain.

I believe that there is a simpler explanation for his anger. To make sense of the dialogue it helps to categorize the sorts of comments doctors make in communicating with patients. An incomplete list would probably look like this:

DOCTORS' CONVERSATION TOOLS:

| | |
|---|---|
| give directions | reassure |
| ask questions | empathize |
| explain | disregard or ignore |
| listen silently | facilitate |
| interrupt | enlist |
| argue | apologize |

comment on the process of the interview

In this case, what the doctor attempted was reassurance. Unfortunately, reassurance often has in it a denial of the patient's perception of reality. It contains a hint of 'things aren't as bad as you think they are.' Or even worse: 'things aren't as bad as you are making them out to be.' A patient's response is likely to be on the order of 'things are every bit as bad as I said, probably worse.' The patient who is the victim of this sort of reassurance not only feels un-reassured, but often feels disregarded, misunderstood, and undervalued. No surprise that he might respond with anger.

What might work better? The strongest therapeutic tool that a physician has available is EMPATHY. Robert Smith and Ruth Hoppe [7] list four emotion-handling skills: naming the emotion, legitimizing it, showing respect for the patient's efforts, and offering support or partnership. We start with a clear statement by the physician that he understands exactly how the patient feels. It sometimes is enough to say just that: "I understand exactly how you feel." However, my preference is to be more specific and say how I think my patient is feeling. Such a statement may be no more than an educated guess. If your assay misses the mark, your patient will usually correct you. In this case you might try: "I can imagine how hard it is for you right now. Not only are you still having this pain, but your physicians seem to be stumped and you aren't sure whether you should continue to stay with them or maybe even go to another place. It must be really scary and uncertain for you right now." My expectation is that a patient like this one would respond with "You're damned tootin!" And he would feel better and be, of all things, reassured.

What if your suggestion fails to satisfy the patient? Sometimes we misdiagnose feelings just as we might misdiagnose anything else. If you suggest to your patient, "I can imagine that you would be frightened by all this" and he responds with a denial and a correction such as. "Not frightened so much as just angry," you can accept the correction and understand him better. "Oh, I see. Not so much frightened as angry. That makes sense to me. I can imagine just how you would feel that way."

Why does your patient feel better? I suppose the central desire most of us have is to be understood. When ill, we suffer from all sorts of symptoms: pain, dyspnea, weakness, nausea, and so on. But universal in illness is the symptom of isolation. We are really all alone with our illnesses. If someone understands how we feel, we are a little bit less alone. We could perceive our efforts at empathy as a treatment for isolation.

Sometimes physicians fear to use empathic statements because they think such statements might suggest even more fearful possibilities to the patient, possibilities that he hasn't yet imagined and now will add to his worries. But I doubt that that ever occurs. Patients have thought of much worse than you would ever suggest. The patient in this interview had considered that his problem hadn't been diagnosed and that perhaps he needed to go elsewhere. He told us just that. Our understanding will not lead him to more fearfulness, quite the contrary.

Finally, you might ask, is there no role at all for reassurance? Yes, there is. Just limit efforts at reassurance to what you can deliver yourself. Reassurances may be as simple as "I will be in to see you later today." Or, "I'm not sure if we can do anything about this tumor, but I will stick with you." Or, "I doubt that I can help you here, but I know a doctor who can and I will arrange for him to come by." Then, you had best be sure to deliver on your promises.

# CAN WE SEE YOUR PATIENT?

Saturday, 1:30 AM, the phone rang.

Dr. A: Hello, this is Dr. Anneberg.

C: This is the clerk at the City General Emergency Room. We have your patient, Anna Stalwart here. Can we have your OK to treat her? Can we see your patient?

A: I don't know. What's the trouble with her? Why is she there? Is there something special about her insurance that leads you to be calling me?

C: She says she's numb on her left side. She has Preak insurance.

A: OK, I see. They only authorize some hospitals in situations that aren't major emergencies. Are you on the Preak list?

C: I don't know. I'll ask her.

A: Wait!

[Long silence]

C: OK, she doesn't know. I think maybe she's been drinking. I'll go ask the head nurse.

A: Wait, please!

[Long silence]

C: OK, I asked the charge nurse. She says we aren't in the Preak system but that we can see your patient if you authorize it.

A: Did I understand that Ms. Stalwart is standing right there?

C: Yes, she is. We didn't want to put her in a booth until we had your permission to treat her.

A: Can you have your nurse or doctor get enough of a look at her to screen her? I need to know if she needs be seen there or can go to another emergency room, one in the HMO she's a member of.

C: No, I'm sorry. We don't do screening. This is the emergency room. The screening clinic is in the medical clinic and only open in the regular day hours.

A: Could your charge nurse just check her?

C: Only if we log her in and treat her like any other patient and then you have to OK it.

A: I see. Can I talk to her?

C: Sure. I'll get her.

[Silence]

S: Hello? This is Anna.

A: Ms. Stalwart? I'm Dr. Anneberg. I thought I was going to talk to the charge nurse. OK, let me tell you that I'm having trouble remembering you. Have I seen you before?

S: Sure; don't you remember me? I saw you a year or so ago. You told me I should lose some weight.

A: Hmm. And how old are you?

S: Twenty nine. I've got Preak insurance.

A: And what's going on now?

S: They don't want to wait on me until they get your permission.

A: Oh, no, I mean what is going on medically? What sort of trouble are you having? How did you decide to go to the emergency room?

S: Oh, I was just driving by with my girl friend. She said that if my arm and leg had been numb I ought to get it seen to. So we stopped off here. They've been numb for two or three days, not all the time, but on and off.

A: I see. Well, Anna, the bad news is that you've gone to the wrong hospital. And you should have called me ahead of time. The Preak people will only pay if you go to the right place after you've called me. So you need to get back in the car with your friend and go to the St. Elsewhere Hospital Emergency Room. Do you know where that is? It's right across the street from my office.

S: Can't they just see to me here since I'm here now? It's not anything very serious, I'm sure.

## DISCUSSION

What an aggravation! To be awakened with this unfortunate administrative problem. And to have to make a medical decision about transfer to another facility without benefit of any sort of screening by competent medical people at the first place!

The doctor is caught in a difficult spot. Probably whatever he does, someone will be dissatisfied, maybe everyone. If he OK's her treatment at the current hospital, the HMO administration will be angry. If he doesn't, there is a risk that she could suffer from the delay in the transfer.

This patient did travel the three miles from City General Hospital to St. Elsewhere where her problem was addressed. She had a strong aroma of alcohol about her; her blood alcohol level was 150 mg/dl. The physical examination was normal and did not clarify her symptoms of numbness of the left arm and leg. She was sent home, told to avoid alcohol, and asked to come to the office to see Dr. A. in three days. She failed to keep the appointment.

Going a step back, it seems possible that she and her friend were both drunk when they presented at the city hospital emergency room. If so, they shouldn't have been returned to the road. A good healthcare system would have followed sensible guidelines and the people in the emergency department would have been concerned about such a hazard. In the end the insurance muddle seems to have prevented us from practicing good medicine or good sense.

# LOTS OF HELP

Dr. L:  Mr. Trout? I'm Dr. Louis. I work with Dr. Berris and he wants me to look you over.  Is this Mrs. Trout?

Mrs. T:  Yes, Doctor, I'm Bill's wife.

Dr. L:  Well, Mr. Trout, if you are comfortable sitting up in bed, I'll move this chair over here.  Mrs. Trout, do you want to take a little time off? Maybe a cup of coffee in the cafeteria? I'll be keeping your husband busy for 45 minutes or so.

Mrs. T:  Doctor, I'd really prefer to stay.

Dr. L:  OK, fine. Mr. Trout, how about telling about this trouble you've been having.

Mrs. T:  He's just not himself, Doctor. He hasn't been well for the last two months.

Dr. L:  OK, what sort of not-well have you been feeling, Mr. Trout?

Mrs. T:  Well, for one thing, he has that terrible cough.

Dr. L:  It would really help me to hear the story from Mr. Trout first and then perhaps you can add comments afterward, Mrs. Trout.

Mrs. T:  All right Doctor; but he never seems to tell doctors how bad he has been feeling.

Dr. L:  Mr. Trout, when do you last recall feeling well?

Mr. T:  Let's see, I was OK at Thanksgiving, wasn't I dear?

Mrs. T:  No Bill, don't you remember? You had that bout with fever and breathing trouble early in November. You never really seemed to recover even after Dr. Smith gave you all those antibiotics.

Dr. L:  And then?

Mrs. T:  Then he just got weaker and weaker. He doesn't eat enough and he used to be a wonderful eater. I bet he's lost 20 pounds.

Dr. L:  What seem to be the most bothersome symptoms to you, Mr. Trout?

Mrs. T:  He seems mostly to complain of that cough. Sometimes he gets those wracking coughing spells that go on and on. He turns all red and I don't know what to do. I don't think the cough has really gone away since all this began last fall.

Dr. L: Mrs. Trout, I really have to ask you to let your husband answer my questions.

Mrs. T: All right, Doctor. I'm sorry.

Dr. L: That's OK. Now, Mr. Trout, if I understand right, you've been sick for about four months with a cough and some shortness of breath and weakness. Your appetite has fallen off and you've lost weight. Is that right?

Mr. T: Yeah, that's all true. I don't have much oomph anymore. My get up and go has got up and went.

Dr. L: Well then, any other symptoms? Pain? Fever? Nausea? Anything else?

Mr. T: I think I had some fever at the start of all this, didn't I, Pearl?

Mrs. T: No, Bill, it wasn't right at the start, but maybe a few months later you had that temperature. That was when Dr. Berris put you on the Bactrim. Then you got so sick to your stomach.

Dr. L: How about pain? Anything hurting?

Mr. T: Not really. Except when I have those coughing spells. Then my whole body aches.

Dr. L: What sort of health problems did you have before last fall?

Mrs. T: He's always been healthy as a horse, doctor. That's why we've been so worried now. Even Dr. Berris is worried. He says Bill isn't himself. He's worried about the chest X-ray too.

Dr. L: Are you a cigarette smoker or a drinker?

Mrs. T: He never was much of a drinker but he used to smoke like a chimney. He quit last fall when the cough started. He smoked more than my brother, and Tom, that's my brother, he smoked plenty.

Dr. L: Any chronic medical problems? High blood pressure? Heart disease? Diabetes? Anything you need to take medicines for?

Mrs. T: No, doctor. He doesn't even take a vitamin.

## DISCUSSION

Is there a doctor in the world who has not experienced an interview such as this? Did you have just this sort of experience yesterday? When asked what is going on, many physicians answer that it is a problem of a "wimpy patient." The fellow just has no spunk. Or they diagnose it as a problem of an overbearing or henpecking wife. The doctors often seem angry with the patient and his spouse.

We might pause a moment to note that this syndrome is almost gender specific. We seldom experience a husband who insists so emphatically in taking over the task of telling his wife's medical story. It is almost always the wife who intervenes. That should give us a hint. Anything so gender specific might reflect a biologic or a social phenomenon. Surely women are bullied every bit as much by their husbands as the converse. But women seldom are replaced by their husbands in telling a story to the doctor.

In our society, the wife is frequently the family communicator. She may have been given or may have assumed the role of talker. This husband may defer to his wife whenever any verbal communication is needed. He may be the strong but very silent type.

Or, she may be the caretaker. She may have the task of caring for any sick person in the family. If so, she is sort of a physician's extender in the family. When she brings her patient to the doctor, she needs to be debriefed. If she isn't heard, she will suffer from collegiate ostracization and will have hurt feelings. I can identify with this syndrome. As a general internist, I refer patients to subspecialists. If I call my consulting cardiologist to see a patient whom I'm having trouble with, I expect him to allow me to tell what I've been going through with this patient. In fact, even if the subspecialist thinks that I am a pretty dumb fellow, unable to diagnose my way out of a paper bag, still he will treat me with respect and listen to my story to be sure that I send him other patients in the future. So we ought to treat this collegiate caretaker politely as she tries to tell us about her patient.

Of course, these are all just conjectures until we have some verification. In this case, a miracle occurred. As the staff physician was struggling, trying to elicit some sort of independent history from his patient, trying to subdue the intervening wife, the door burst open and an orderly announced that he had come to take the patient for a chest X-ray the patient's admitting physician had requested. The staff physician was glad of a reprieve; that left him alone with his patient's wife. In a stroke of genius, Dr. Louis asked Mrs. Trout "How have things been going for you?"

She burst into tears and after sobbing several minutes explained that her only brother was dying of lung cancer. She was sure that he would die soon. Now she thought her husband too probably had lung cancer and would die. She would be all alone. She was grieving her losses. After she talked about her fears, her vision of being left all alone, and her sadness, she was able to converse more quietly. When her husband returned from the radiology department, she remained quiet while he told his story. She no longer seemed to need to intervene.

What can we conclude? I believe the best analysis is that Dr. Louis had two patients. One suffered from cough, fatigue and anorexia. The other suffered from anxiety, near panic, and a great deal of grief. Of the two, the one who most needed to be heard was the second. Indeed, if Dr. Louis had been called to the emergency ward and told that he needed to see two patients in two separate rooms, one suffering from months of fatigue, cough, and weight loss, the other suffering from panic and overwhelming grief, it would probably have been obvious that the latter needed attention first.

In this interview the problem was that only one person was identified as a patient. Dr. Louis had trouble recognizing the existence of the second even though she was clamoring for his attention. This situation is not rare. Sometimes the distressed "other patient" is noted as a relative who cannot seem to hear explanations about the sick or dying patient. "No matter how I explain to him, he doesn't understand what is happening to his son." Such an "un-understanding, unteachable" relative should trigger our suspicions that we have another person who needs be understood, not lectured to. It is not uncommon that we have more than one patient on our hands at one time, more than one person needing our help, and that perhaps the one not identified as a patient may be the only one we can help.

# JUST A COLD

Mr. George:  Thanks for seeing me on short notice, Doc. I wouldn't come in if I wasn't nearly dead.

Doctor X:  Oh? How are you feeling bad?

G:  I've been sick all week and I'm scheduled to fly to Portland this weekend.

X:  What sort of symptoms?

G:  Mostly a sinus infection. I can't breathe and I've got this yellow stuff I keep blowing out my nose.

X:  You can't breathe?

G:  Nah. My sinuses are so stuffed up, like now, I can hardly breathe on the left side of my nose.

X:  How is it with your mouth open?

G:  That's fine. But I can't go around like some kind of fish, you know.

X:  OK, then. Stuffy head, nasal drainage, what else?

G:  That's it. That's enough. Usually I get these colds and they're gone in one or two days. This one I've had all week.

X:  I see. Any other symptoms? Cough? Fever? Anything else?

G:  Nah. Maybe a tickle in my throat; I cough once or twice.  No big deal though.

X:  O.K., let's take a look at you. Hop up here on the examination table and slip off your shirt.

X:  Mr. George, the exam is entirely normal. All you've got is a cold. Take one of the over-the-counter decongestants, Dristan or Contact for example.  Maybe a couple of aspirins. We'll see you for your physical in six months.

G:  You mean you aren't going to give me something for this? I gotta go out of town in three days and I can't still be sick then.

X:  Yes, sometimes we use an antibiotic, but you aren't sick enough to make that worthwhile.

G: What? I'm sick as I want to be. What is this? I'm not sick enough? What's going on? Is this because I'm capitation in Compli-Care? They tell you to save a few bucks by not prescribing penicillin?

X: That doesn't have anything to do with it. I treat you just like patients who pay right up front.

G: Hey! I pay plenty for this insurance, Doc, and I don't see how I'm getting my money's worth.


# DISCUSSION

I'd begin by focusing on the doctor's explanation of the "negative" examination and of the diagnosis, prognosis, and therapy. This doctor explained almost nothing. The patient is always eager to know what has happened to him, what may happen if he does nothing further therapeutically, and what the doctor is suggesting that he do. Even patients with trivial illness may need major explanations and one should not assume that a trivial illness requires only a cursory discussion.

In fact, as a rule of thumb, you might assume that the extent of explanation needed is inversely proportionate to the severity and danger of the illness.

This doctor was rushed and understandably impatient with a man who had insisted on being fitted into a busy schedule for a trivial illness, and who expected miraculous cures. Unfortunately, as in 'haste makes waste,' impatience slows things down.

What might the physician have done?

He might have said something like this:

Dr. X: I think you have a viral infection of your upper respiratory tract. It involves the nose and the lining of the respiratory system, probably the sinuses too, as you suggested. We can call that a "cold" if we wish but even a common cold can be quite bothersome and make life really miserable for you. The trouble is that there is no useful therapy beyond some symptom relief. We usually suggest one of the decongestants that are available over the counter and are really as useful as anything we can prescribe. Then, intense humidity—steam—helps some. If you fly into Portland and are more stuffed up on landing, or if your ears are painful, you might need some intense humidity.

The trouble is that there is no effective treatment or cure for these infections. We just have to wait it out.

G: You mean that you aren't going to give me an antibiotic?

X: I'm glad you asked that. It would probably be a mistake to treat you with an antibiotic. They have no effect at all on viruses and this is almost certainly a viral cold. The antibiotics often do damage. For example, they can cause really nasty and persistent diarrhea. I think that would be a bad choice.

G: You mean I gotta just wait it out?

X: I'm afraid so. Now I do want you to keep an eye out for complications. Even viral illnesses can develop into something worse. For example, if you start coughing up a lot of dark green stuff or get fevers over 101 or chest pain or shortness of breath or start turning blue, I'd like you to come back in to see me.

G: You bet I would. If I start turning blue, you'll be the first to know. OK, Doc. Let's see. You want me to take Dristan and steam and come back if I'm worse or just not better in a couple of weeks, right?

X: Right.


A few important points:

1. The doctor used the same terminology as the patient, sinus infection in his explanation. The patient's diagnostic hypothesis, his explanatory model for his illness, was sinus infection. Some attention should be paid to that theory in the doctor's explanation. At the least, the doctor should let the patient know that he has considered that diagnosis.[8]

2. The doctor and the patient repeat each other's phrases at the end of the interaction. "Just wait it out" and "Right" demonstrate that they are on the same wavelength.

3. The doctor gives a reason for withholding antibiotics and emphasizes that this is in the patient's best interest. Again, the doctor and the patient are on the same team.

# ADMISSION INTERVIEW

Dr. A: Mr. Smythe, I'm Dr. Anthony. I'm the medical resident this month and Dr. Miller asked me to see you. He will be by later. How are you doing?

Mr. S: Fine. Much better now.

Dr. A: Well, I need to review your entire history, so perhaps you can tell me what brought you to Presbyterian Hospital.

Mr. S: I thought I ought to see one of the cardiologists who does surgery. I figured he'd be best for me.

Dr. A: Why a surgeon? Why not a medical cardiologist?

Mr. S: Well, the medical guys don't do anything. If you need something done to you it better be by a surgical cardiologist.

Dr. A: Was there something wrong with your heart?

Mr. S: I figured there was. I've had two heart catheterizations and Dr. Sheridan does cardiograms every chance he gets. I imagine that's just so he can charge me for them. He and Snyder have me taking about five different heart medicines. I pay more for those pills than I used to pay for a car.

Dr. A: I'm confused. Do you think that Dr. Sheridan only does cardiograms so he can charge you for them?

Mr. S: Oh, not really. He's a great guy, Sheridan. I like to kid him a little. He and I used to play golf some together. That was before I had heart trouble but I bet he still plays. I like him better than the guy I had taking care of me before.

Dr. A: Who was that?

Mr. S: Buckhortz. He must have been before your time. He's been dead more than ten years.

Dr. A: Oh. OK, let's get back to your heart. Have you been having pain?

Mr. S: You bet. I've had angina for five or six years. When it started, Sheridan was away in Palm Springs or somewhere, playing golf, I imagine. He thinks he's Nicklaus. Anyway, Fineman started me out on Inderal and nitro. By the time Sheridan got back I was out of the hospital and back at work. He said that he'd have to schedule all his vacations for when I got sick. I wouldn't be surprised if he could; he goes away so much.

Dr. A: Do you have any other heart symptoms? Shortness of breath? Swelling of your legs? Cough? Palpitations?

Mr. S: Just when I see a pretty girl. Did you see the nurse who checked me in here? I wish I was thirty years younger.

Dr. A: What? You get short of breath when you see a pretty woman?

Mr. S: No, just kidding. I don't have any of those things. If it wasn't for the heart pain, I'd be OK.

Dr. A: What medicines are you taking? Anything but the Inderal and the nitroglycerine?

Mr. S: That's it. Plus a Dyazide and two Cardizams. And I take some vitamins, of course. Then sometimes I take a few aspirins. And I use one of those herbal laxatives sometimes but that's natural.

Dr. A: Smoke?

Mr. S: Not anymore. When Fineman gave me the Inderal he lectured me about cigarettes and I decided it was better me than them.

Dr. A: Drink?

Mr. S: What? Alcohol? Sure, but not like I used to. I'll take an occasional drink but just social. I don't drink that much.

Dr. A: Any operations or hospitalizations in the past?

Mr. S: Just my tonsils when I was a kid. They used to take out everyone's tonsils then. And Snyder did the two heart caths. That's when he decided I had spasm and didn't need an operation. I thought this time I was ready but he says not yet.

Dr. A: So why are you still here in a hospital?

Mr. S: Well, the more they did, the tireder I got. It just looked like I couldn't manage at home if I wasn't stronger.

Dr. A: OK, I want to ask you about your family and then review some other areas and then do an examination. I think I've got the main problem down now.

## DISCUSSION

It helps to consider the sort of communications we hear from our patients, especially in answer to our "how are you feeling?", "what sort of trouble have you been having?", or "what brought you to see me today?" And then consider what responses are most helpful to us.

What the patient is talking about:

symptoms
physical signs of disease
laboratory results
diagnoses
theories of pathophysiology
plans
tangential sequence (farther afield each utterance)
circumstantial sequence (events surrounding illness)
   n.b. saga of medical care (SOMC) = medical circumstances.
miscellaneous

Nothing the patient ever says is meaningless; everything he or she says is of significance. It helps to assume that whatever the patient says has to do with him and with now.

However, it is also true that not everything the patient says is equally useful to the doctor. Above all, what we want to hear about are symptoms. Symptoms are the gold of interviewing and just like the apocryphal story about the famous bank robber, Willie Sutton, who, when asked why he robbed banks, supposedly replied, "Because that's where the money is," we should go where the gold is. First of all, the patient cannot be mistaken about symptoms. He may lie or deny a symptom or forget or embellish it, but he can't be mistaken in the same way that he may be mistaken about a diagnosis. If he says that he has pain in his leg, that is what he has. But if he says that he is suffering from sciatica, he may be mistaken. He may not be the clever diagnostician that he thinks he is, or he may be quoting another doctor to you. That doctor might not be so clever a diagnostician, or the patient may have misunderstood his other doctor, but he can't be wrong about the symptom. And the symptom can be discussed sensibly; you can ask questions about it for clarification. As our legal friends might say, the symptom is subject to cross examination; it is not hearsay evidence. We should consider symptoms to be the primary data we solicit in the history. Everything else is of secondary importance in our effort to reach a correct diagnosis.

This patient provides everything but symptoms. He seems to be under the impression that to talk to doctors you need to employ doctor talk, and that such doctor talk consists of diagnoses, treatments, and test results—just like the way doctors talk to him. I call this the saga of medical care. It makes a good popular magazine article, dramatizing the workings of the medical system, but never leads to any diagnoses except those already made. If the doctor is to do doctoring, she has to coax the patient gently from the saga of medical care to describing his symptoms and the illness itself.

Not easy! The doctor may find it hard because he is convinced that he needs to hear all the events of medical care to know where to go next. If the doctor realizes that he must shift the patient's emphasis, the task is still difficult. It is all too easy to make the patient feel unheard or bullied, angering him or hurting his feelings.

Dr. A: Mr. S., what sort of symptoms were you having?
Mr. S: I'm trying to tell you, if you will just listen!

If, as in this interaction, we begin with a patient who talks freely but omits symptoms, we may inadvertently silence him just by trying to redirect him to a symptomatic history. As we try to direct the patient more to what we think we needto hear, he may become stymied, feel limited and give up. Then we end up with a high-doctor-control interview, a problem just as bad as the one we started with.

There is no easy solution. When confronted with an interviewing problem, the approach that works most often is to explain our problem to the patient and enlist his help. "I'm having a little difficulty here. I understand the story you have told me about your illness and the various diagnoses and treatments and tests. But I would like to understand more about the specific symptoms you have had. How have you been feeling? What ways have you been feeling ill?" Perhaps surprisingly, most patients understand the word "symptom" and can provide symptoms when asked, "What sort of symtoms have you been having?"

# MAY I ASK YOU A REALLY STUPID QUESTION?

Frank Malone, a 76 year old retired tailor who was well except for a controlled seizure disorder, became ill on Friday afternoon with chills and cough. His wife, Ellen, called me and found that I was off for the weekend but my on-call colleague suggested that Frank go to the emergency room. Frank's son came to drive him, and rather than take him across town to my usual hospital, he took his father to a closer hospital, unfortunately not one where I practiced. A physician in the emergency room diagnosed pneumonia. The patient was admitted to the inpatient service, and a new internist was found to care for him.

Returning to work on Monday, I discovered the events of the weekend. I called Frank's hospital room and talked with his wife who said that Dr. Smith was caring for Frank but that she had yet to meet Dr. Smith. I promised to come out and visit Frank the next day or the day after. Thus it was Wednesday, five days after Frank had become ill, that I drove across the city and looked in on my patient, assigned to Dr. Smith, but actually being cared for by his colleague, Dr. Brown. Frank was feeling "terrible" and was quite warm with a recorded temperature of 104 despite antibiotic therapy for the last five days. He had decreased breath sounds at the right lung base, a finding that conformed to the radiology report of a right lower-lobe pneumonia. I was puzzled by Frank's failure to respond to the second generation cephalosporin. I explained the problem to Frank and Ellen and wrote a note in the chart suggesting that perhaps a different antibiotic might be better. I wondered about an aspiration pneumonia but both Frank and Ellen insisted that there had been no recent seizures.

Dr. P: I'm really puzzled. It looks as if Dr. Brown has been treating Frank with an adequate antibiotic, yet he still has a high fever. That suggests that there is something going on we don't understand. Did Frank have a seizure in the few days before he got sick with chills and coughing?

E: No, he hasn't had a seizure since that one about six months ago. He had been doing really well.

P: Well I must admit that I am puzzled. Something has him sick here and we aren't finding it.

[Pause]

E: Excuse me, Doctor, but could I ask you a really stupid question?

P: Sure. Besides, you know there isn't such a thing as a dumb question, although there probably are some dumb answers.

E: Well, it's just that his grandchildren got him a birthday present last month, a cockatiel.

P: A cockatiel! Right!

E: Yes, and it's a terrible mess. It has all this dander and keeps scattering feathers and everything all over. I think maybe we ought to get rid of it.

[I got up and walked around the bed to give Ellen a hug.]

P: That's it. Frank has parrot fever. We need to switch antibiotics.

E: You mean there is such a thing as parrot pneumonia?

P: Yes. And I would never have thought to ask you a question about it. How wonderful that you thought to tell me!

E: Well, it's just that it is such a messy bird. We thought maybe we ought to get it out of the house.


## DISCUSSION

Why do patients and their families feel so reluctant to tell us what we most need to hear? How do we prepare the ground so they are more easily able to do just that? Surely this patient's wife was hesitant to say anything, even though she had the critical new information. She didn't know how important the new family bird was, but her shyness probably stems from her shyness with doctors in general.

And are physicians failing in their needs to communicate with one another? What would the result of more politeness between doctors be? In this case, the physician who had taken over the care of this patient had not made any effort to contact the primary care physician, answering Ellen's requests that he involve Dr. P. with "We usually send them a copy of the discharge summary."

I think perhaps these two communication problems are related. If we indicate a willingness to hear from one source of information, perhaps we will also be able to hear from another. This conversation surely qualifies as a minor miracle, and I was not aware of having done anything myself to elicit the key piece of information. Yet we can communicate a willingness to listen. Surely a doctor's unwillingness to listen can be perceived by patient or spouse and then will curtail any useful conversation.

This woman had not thought the new doctor was eager to talk with her and her own shyness kept her from broaching what she thought would be viewed as a foolish question, asking whether they should get rid of the bird. Only when her familiar physician appeared did she hesitantly raise the subject.

And I believe that doctors are not treating each other with much politeness. I think that they used to do better. Twenty five years ago, when I was new in medicine, the AMA had a "code of ethics" that was more a code of etiquette. It dealt with how doctors should talk to each other, how they should relate to each other. We now realize that medical ethics have much more to do with how doctors treat patients but we seem to have forgotten our manners in dealing with each other. Surely a physician caring for a patient who usually is cared for by another doctor should communicate with his colleague. Good manners, good medicine, and legal necessities argue for such conversations.

However, this case might be an exception to prove the rule. I suspect that if Dr. Brown had called me on Monday or Tuesday, I would have been reassured that my patient was in good hands and that appropriate therapy was being carried out. Perhaps I wouldn't have made the trip on Wednesday and would not have heard that single most important, 'really stupid' question. What was the question anyway? Was it, should we get rid of the bird? Maybe it was, would knowing that we have a debris-scattering cockatiel help you right now?

Changing the antibiotic to tetracycline did the trick. Frank defervesced immediately and he was home in three days. His chlamydial antibodies rose dramatically over the next three weeks. The bird had similarly high antibodies when tested by its veterinarian. The vet did call me promptly.

How did I feel about all this? Yes, I was affronted by Dr. Brown's failure to contact me in the first place. Yes, I did feel great joy to discover the bird story, and even more joy that I was the one to make the discovery. Yes, I took fiendish joy at being able to inform Dr. Brown, and yes I gloated; I have to admit it, I absolutely gloated at my little triumph.

# GONE MISSING

Dr. Ham:  Hello, I'm Dr. Ham. Are you Dr. Brown's patient?

Mrs. Briskett:  Yes, I am. I'm Helen Briskett.

H:  Your name again?

B:  Briskett, Helen Briskett.

H:  And how old are you?

B:  I'm 90. And this is only my second time in the hospital ever.

H:  Are you from Denver?

B:  Well, I was raised in Wyoming. My family were ranchers. Then I had one child, but she died at 37 from a heart attack. I raised my two grandchildren myself.

H:  And you live in Denver now?

B:  Yes, there is a woman who cares for me.

H:  How long have you been in the hospital?

B:  I came in last Monday. I hadn't felt well for three weeks, but I don't like to go to doctors.

H:  You hadn't been feeling well? What sort of symptoms did you have? How were you feeling poorly?

B:  Well, I had a cough and I kept coughing up yellow cold. And I was tired all the time.

H:  I see. Cough and tired. Anything else? Fever?

B:  I didn't think so. But when I got here they told me I was 101.

H:  Then cough, tired, and fever. Anything else? Any other problems?

B:  No. Except that I have a lot of allergies so I can't take medicines. That's kept me strong and well.

H:  Can you tell me about your family?

B:  There wasn't much. Just my daughter, and she died. My parents lived to be old, like me.

H:  That's a healthy family then. Lucky. Any other problems you haven't mentioned?

B:  No.  Except that I couldn't breathe well yesterday. Usually I do all right. I live near Cheesman park and I have friends. We play bridge. I used to play golf and I only gave it up about a year ago.

# DISCUSSION

We all fail to concentrate from time to time. But what we most have to offer our patients is our attention, so we must strive to remain conscious. In this fragment of an interview, the most striking flaw is the doctor's failure to respond to the information about the patient's most important life loss. She lost her only daughter, has mentioned it twice, and the doctor missed the significance of that loss. The doctor even suggested that she and her family had been blessed with good luck in health matters after the patient had again told him of her most grievous loss.

Later on, asked what he had been thinking, the doctor said, "Oh yeah, I guess she had mentioned that." Still it didn't seem a serious oversight to him. What pain is there in life that equates to the loss of a child? And an only child at that! This woman had told us, twice, of the worst thing that had ever happened to her.

What is an appropriate response to hearing of the worst thing that ever happened to someone? Surely recognition of that fact. The 1960's flower children popularized comments like "Oh, wow!" Trite and non-specific, but how appropriate! The doctor could say "Oh, wow! That sounds terrible. That must be the worst thing that could ever happen to a person." And, of course, the technique again is empathy—some effort to let the patient know that you understand how she feels.

This doctor may be concentrating on a physical problem and surely wants to help his patient. But the doctor must know that he can help his patients on several levels. The interview itself, the listening, the examination can all be of help, truly curative of soul sickness.[9, 10]

Sometimes we neglect opportunities for empathetic response because we are unfamiliar with the technique, other times because we missed the significance of the patient's message. But we ought to keep alert to really painful messages and we ought to listen up if we hear the same thing twice. It is probably important. Otherwise, it is just as if we are not there during the interview, gone missing.

# A STERN PERSON
(Thanks to Dr. Robert Bosworth)

Dr. Bosworth: Hello, I'm Dr. Bosworth. Are you Ms. Nugent?

Ms. N: (stern-visaged woman, dressed in black, with gloves and hat) Yes, but before we start, I have a few questions.

B: OK. Go ahead.

N: Are you a diagnostician?

B: Well, I am an internist. We consider ourselves to be diagnosticians, yes.

N: And how many diagnoses do you make?

B: Well, I see about fifteen people a day. And I probably make one or two diagnoses for each. So, I suppose I make about 25 diagnoses a day.

N: And of those 25, how many are correct?

B: Well, a lot are tentative and later turn out to be something else. I suppose about 50% are correct.

N: In that case, I am in the wrong place. (She rises, leaves the office, and is never seen there again.)

## DISCUSSION

Dr. Bosworth, a cheerful person who is not easily ruffled, recalls this interaction as one of the strangest of his 30 years of clinical practice. He was bemused as he told me of it. He says he was captivated by the woman's style and thought nothing could really be done differently. Indeed, as a humorous clinical vignette, perhaps nothing could make it better. However as a chance to begin a therapeutic relationship and a doctor-patient interaction, surely it went badly. What could be done differently?

We all have experiences where we wish we had said something different. After conversations we think of what we wish we had said. But if we are alert to the existence of a conversational pitfall, we can gently stop the process and then introduce other permutations. For example, after this wonderful initial conversation, as the patient was leaving the room, the doctor could say "Just a minute!" The doctor could ask the patient to come back. "Before you go, may I ask a favor? Would you also answer a few questions for me?" Surely the patient, intrigued by the approach, would come back. Then it is time to say that her approach had interested you, that you knew at the time that you were giving very incomplete answers to very complex questions, and that you were interested to know what led her to approach you with such queries. After all, an important part of our job is to be the interrogator. Surely we should not find it hard to turn the tables back in our usual direction.

Dr. Geoff Gordon says that he likes to identify the 900 pound gorilla that is sitting on his chest. He thinks that this patient has a major concern and that we don't have to make random guesses about her concerns but that we might try something like:

B: It sounds like you're concerned that I might not have enough expertise or skill to take care of you.

Such a remark may be enough to bring her into the interaction in a more effective fashion.

This case also illustrates a patient's misapprehensions about what doctors can do. So it provides an opportunity for patient education, not just about her specific illness, but about our roles and our limitations. Viewed as such an opportunity, she indeed was one who got away.

# PHONE CALLS FROM
# THE EMERGENCY ROOM

Dr. FP, at home, is often awakened at night by phone calls from the local emergency departments. For instance,

I. FP: Hello?

Dr. Amphioxus: Hi, I'm Leonard here in the emergency room. We have a patient who has no assigned staff doctor. Will you take him on?

FP: OK. Tell me about him.

Dr. A: He's been taking a bunch of drugs and has chest pain. What do you want to do?

II. FP: Hello?

Dr. B: Hello, I'm Dr. Bezoar. I'm in the Presbyterian Hospital Emergency Room and I have Mrs. Chaplip here. She's 84, fell over today, and can't move. She feels fine otherwise. She's on Lasix, dig, quinidine, Zantac, Xanax, and vitamins. Her labs are all OK except that the glucose is 154. The chest X-ray is normal and the cardiogram shows just some mild T changes. I thought we ought to keep her here overnight and see how she feels in the morning, OK?

III. FP: Hello?

Dr. Denture: Hi, this is Jim Denture. I'm the staff doctor in the St. Luke's Emergency Department today. I've got your patient, John Always here. He has pain in his right elbow. There's no dyspnea, no chest pain, no radiation to the back or the neck, no nausea, no dizziness. He says he feels strong and has a good appetite and that his bowels moved regularly today. He has no urinary pain and no frequency, no fever or chills, no rashes or faintness. He has been OK in the past except for some knee surgery and a tonsillectomy. His family all seem healthy. On exam the HEENT reveal normal fundi and good EOMs. He's got a slightly deviated nasal septum. His neck and lymph nodes are OK. There are no rales or rhonchi and his back doesn't show any scoliosis. His PMI is in the MCL and I don't hear any murmurs or rubs. The abdomen is OK except for some vague epigastric tenderness. He has normal bowel sounds, no edema, good reflexes. The SMA 72 is normal except that his uric acid is 7.9 and his CBC shows a MCV of 101 even though his H and H are normal. The chest X-ray was OK and his cardiogram fine, I think, but I've asked the medical resident to check it out when he finishes in the unit. The UA was stable and the gram stain didn't show anything. I was wondering if you thought we ought to get a CT or not.

IV. FP: Hello?

Dr. Shortway: Hi, is this Dr. Platt? I'm Norman Shortway, the intern in the St. Joseph E.R. I have your patient Paul Bunyan here. Are you awake enough for me to tell you about him?

FP: What? Oh yeah. Let me write down those names. OK, you're Shortway and he's Bunyan. Go on.

S: Well, he's 63, usually well, and now sick for three days. He's got a cough, bringing up brown sputum, and has some pleuritic pain over the right lateral chest. He smokes three packs a day and drinks about four ounces of vodka daily. The rest of the history seems unremarkable. He has a fever of 102 degrees, pulse 120, BP 175/110, and a respiratory rate of 32. The only real findings are a dry mouth and some rales at the right lateral and anterior chest. I went ahead and got a few labs. The chest X-ray shows an infiltrate in the right middle lobe. He's a little hypoxic with a pO2 of 52 so I put him on some nasal oxygen. The sputum shows a lot of polys and some Gram positive diplococci. I'm waiting for the ECG and CBC and 'lytes but I went up and looked at the sputum smear myself. I think he has a pneumococcal pneumonia. He's kind of sick so I'd like to bring him in and treat him with IV penicillin unless you think a cephalosporin would be better. What do you think?

FP: Bless you.

# DISCUSSION

I. Too little. Who is the doctor anyway? Are you surprised that calls like this really happen? I am always amazed and wonder what the caller expects me to do. Of course we get similar calls from non-physicians, for example, nursing home staff, much more often. That represents a growing and more important problem.

II. Did we miss something? Where was the physical examination? What is the diagnosis? If the doctor assumes that this patient represents some sort of a placement problem, he needs the help of the social service, but this patient still needs a doctor to ferret out her problem.

The old truism says that the three keys to correct therapy are diagnosis, diagnosis, and diagnosis. To reach a correct diagnosis we need at least an appropriate history and the physical examination.

III. Too much. Perhaps we could breed Dr. Amphioxus to Dr. Denture and get the right mixture. Again, no amount of laboratory testing can replace a little careful thought about the diagnostic possibilities.

IV. Perfect.

## MY SUGGESTIONS FOR NIGHT ER
## CALLS TO ATTENDINGS

1. Be sure the person on the other end of the phone is awake.
2. Be brief.
3. Identify yourself and the hospital.
4. Use standard sequence for reports: history (Hx), physical exam (PE), lab and X-ray, diagnosis (Dxs), plans.
5. Be sure to have your own observations, especially vital signs.
6. Tell only positive pertinent features of the Hx and PE. Nobody can really listen to the long presentations that we are taught in medical school. No one really listened even there. Your phone audience will fall asleep again. It also helps the listener to have a clearly identified chief complaint early on in the story.
7. Decide what you think Dxs are and what you want to do before you call the attending.

# HOW SMART ARE YOU DOCTOR?

Mr. Louis: Good to see you, Doctor. How are you doing?

Dr. Fred: Not bad, Bob. I'm getting through my day. How are you?

L: I bet you're doing a lot better than that. After all, you are a smart man. I can tell. What is your IQ anyway? Don't you have to be over 120 just to get into medical school?

F: I don't know, Bob. We didn't even have to take any such tests when I went to medical school.

L: OK, but still you have to be plenty smart. What do you think you are? 140? More?

F: Who knows. I was probably smart as a young man, but now I'm older and lucky if I can find my way to work in the morning.

L: I doubt it. I bet you have to be plenty smart to do your work. You have a lot of complicated cases, don't you Doctor?

F: Too complicated sometimes.

L: No, that couldn't be true. Seriously, what do you think your IQ is?

F: Bob, I really don't know. Can I pick a number?

L: Sure.

F: How about 200?

L: Now, I think you're kidding.

F: You're right. OK, why don't we find out about you. How have you been doing?

L: Not bad, Doctor. Pretty good, I'd say, for the shape I'm in.

F: Any pain? Trouble breathing? Swelling? Any troubles at all?

L: Nope. I've had a good month. Only used two nitros and just in case, like you told me. You said, "Why not take them before you do something so you don't get pain?" So that's what I do.

After some more discussion of the patient's health issues, review of his cardiac and pulmonary status, an examination of the related areas, and plans for the future, the doctor bid the patient adieu.

As he was leaving the room, his patient told him:

L: I've moved back in with my wife again.

I was the puzzled doctor in this conversation. I thought about this last message for three seconds. I had no idea that my patient had not been living with his wife. But now time pressures felt heavy. I repeated my goodbye and we agreed that the patient would return in two months.

## DISCUSSION

This seems a quaint sort of opening conversation. What do you do with the patient's inquiries that seem pointed at you but are not the usual sort of "How's the family?" queries. How are we to place these inquiries? What do they mean?

When in doubt, the best strategy is probably to ask the patient. "What was that all about?" "What is the new sudden interest in your doctor's IQ?" Unfortunately, when asked, later on in the conversation, this patient answered by denying any specific significance, just idle curiosity. Then, feeling that he might have transgressed, he apologized for passing the boundary of good manners. Nothing more was learned.

So, what might one guess?

My favorite rule of thumb for strange medical conversational side-trips is that the patient is always talking about himself and about right now. If your patient tells you a long story about something that happened to his uncle ten years ago, your first guess should be that he is really asking you about himself right now. What in the story about his uncle pertains to his current situation? And in this dialogue about the doctor's intelligence, I would suggest first assuming that the patient is asking something that pertains to him and to now. Such as, "Are you smart enough to understand what is happening to me right now?" With that guess, the doctor might hazard a suggestion: "Are you wondering if I will be smart enough to understand just what is happening to you right now?"

Of course, I missed this message completely. I was finished with my patient, in a hurry to get to the next person whom I had already kept waiting too long. Once he hinted of the problem he and his wife were having, I might have, if I understood the question, answered, "Not smart enough to help you."

Another doctor suggested that this strange interchange was an example of a transference phenomenon. William Zinn [11] defines transference, as Freud did originally, as a process in which individuals displace patterns of behavior and emotional reactions that originated through interaction with significant figures in their childhood onto other persons in their current lives. Does that concept help any here? I don't think so. I think this case is really an example of the bizarre turns that conversation takes, especially when the tale teller is unsure about whether he really wants to tell you the story.

I didn't have a clue what this conversation was about until I thought about it for days. Even then no solution presented itself. It wasn't until I discussed the interchange with a colleague a week later, and she asked me, "What are you going to do?" that I realized that I could still do something.

I phoned the patient. Our conversation was something like this:

F: Bob? This is Doctor Fred.

L: Oh. How you doing Doc?

F: Fine, Bob. But I have been thinking about our conversation when you were here last and I realized that I don't really understand much about what's been going on at home for you. Would you like to come in and talk with me about it?

L: Oh. That's nice of you to call, Doc. I think things are going pretty good now. I don't think I have to come by right now. How about I'll just tell you next time I'm in.

F: OK, Bob. Are you sure?

L: Yeah, sure, doc. Thanks for calling.


Well, I'm not sure that helped any. And I do wish I had been fast enough to think through his questions the first time. Maybe I'll get another chance another time.

# EMERGENCY DEPARTMENT CONVERSATION

## I. PERSONAL CONNECTION

Dr. Ed:  Hello!  What sort of trouble are you having?

Mr. Mangrum:  I've got pain in my chest. I feel awful. I felt as if my pores had opened up and my soul was seeping through.

E:  OK, how long has this been going on?

M:  Not too long, Doc, maybe an hour or two. I was sitting in a White Spot on Colfax and I got so I couldn't breathe right so I went out and sat on the curb and someone called the paramedics.

E:  Any other symptoms? Just the pain and dyspnea?

M:  Just pain and not breathing. Are you the doctor here?

E:  Yeah. OK, let me listen to your chest here. Take a couple of deep breaths. (He listens with his stethoscope while the patient moves his chest up and down, moving very little air). OK, let me listen to your heart. (He listens.) I'll have the nurse hook you up to our monitor. (He goes out the door.)

R:  Hello, I'm Richard. I've got to take a cardiogram on you. You doing OK?

M:  I don't know. Some doctor was just here, I think. He didn't tell me what he thought.

[Discussion follows conversation III]

## II. UNDERSTANDING

Dr. F:  Hello, I'm Dr. Fredericks. I just got a look at your ECG. I think there might be some subendocardial ischemia. I think we better tube you up to the unit and hold you there for obs for a while. OK?

Mr. Mangrum: You're not the same doctor I saw before, are you? What do you mean "obs"?

Dr. F: Nothing serious. We'll just hook you up to the monitor, start an IV, give you some O's and do some enzymes. We'll know more in a day or two.

Mr. M: Enzymes? What? Are they serious? Wait a minute!

(Dr. F. is already out the door.)

[Discussion follows conversation III]

## III. (A NEW PATIENT) EMPATHY

Dr. G: Hi, I'm Dr. Gross. I need to hear about your trouble that brought you to the emergency department today.

Mr. Frank: This is the fourth time I've been here with my troubles. You look awfully young to be a doctor. You're not an intern, are you?

G: Yeah, I am. I'm a surgery intern and I'm covering the ED tonight. What sort of trouble are you having?

F: I've been having pains in my gut, dreadful pains that double me up, and nobody seems to think there is anything wrong with me. They seem to think it's all in my head.

G: OK, tell me more about this belly pain. Exactly where is it?

F: It's right here on the right side, above my belly button. I get it and I can't hardly walk or talk. Then it passes and I'm all right again. I had it an hour ago and they had to carry me over here in an ambulance and now I'm about normal again.

G: Any other symptoms along with the pain? Nausea or vomiting? Trouble with your urine or bowels?

F: No, it's just the pain. I'm beginning to wonder if I'm crazy. Maybe I ought to go see a mental doctor.

G: Well, let me look at your stomach. (He pulls up the patient's gown and does an abdominal exam.) Now, roll over. I'm going to check your rectum. (He helps the patient over onto his side, puts on a glove, and does a rectal exam.) OK, I agree with you, everything looks fine now.

F: I can't understand how it can hurt so much and then be fine again so fast. I'm afraid something awful is happening and no one seems to be able to figure it out.

G: Well, let me check some blood studies. I'll have the technician draw some blood and we'll be back in a while.

## DISCUSSION

We are often pressed for time, nowhere more than in emergency medicine. But that is not an excuse for failure to satisfy conversational needs. In fact, it is more reason for precise use of conversational tools. We do not have time for slipshod work.

There are several key steps in any medical encounter. They include forming a personal connection with the patient, understanding his story, and letting him know that you understand his feelings and accept him as a person.

Personal connections are begun with the usual steps of polite behavior such as greetings, handshakes, eye contact, trading of names, concern for comfort, privacy, and modesty. One of the strongest devices for forming rapid personal connection is the use of names. The patient's name gives you a handle and a control. Your name gives the same to your patient. It is not meaningless that the Old West term for name was 'handle.' Now we hear that term on citizen band radios. If I give you my name, you have my handle and can hold on to me. I become manageable. We should use that powerful device. Even in a brief interaction, we should use the patient's name several times and we must be sure the patient has our name. A business card or a prescription sheet with name clearly and largely written may help but in a pinch you can write your name down for the patient on his sleeve or on the sheet.

Mr. Mangrum never had the benefit of any real connection with his physician. He felt and was disconnected. And he desperately needed information. No one really took time to educate him. In fact, our technical jargon confuses and frightens if we do nothing to interpret it.

In our work we need to understand the patient's story. Then we must tell it back to him so that he knows we understood and so that we can learn where we have gone astray. We need to tell the patient what we think is going wrong, what we propose doing, and what might be the outcome if we do or if we don't follow our plans. And, of course, we need to ask the patient what he understands us to be telling him. Then we must take the opportunity to correct misunderstandings. All that takes a little time but it takes a lot more time to make up for misunderstandings later.

Then we need to let the patient know that we understood how he was feeling emotionally as well as physically. That sense of being understood is the most health-giving awareness we can try to impart. Empathy is our most powerful therapeutic tool. Dr. Gross, for example, might have taken advantage of the obvious opportunity for empathy with Mr. Frank. He could have said: "I can imagine how puzzling it is for you to have such terrific pain and then all of a sudden feel just fine. I can see why you would be puzzled and worry."

That isn't any miraculous psychological insight; Mr. Frank had just said as much himself. But in letting the patient know that we understand how he feels, we are 'getting with' him and the comfort from such a step is enormous.

Mr. Frank provided another good opportunity for empathy that Dr. Gross might have taken advantage of. When the patient commented on Dr. Gross looking young, the physician could have responded "Yes, I do look young. Are you wondering if I am experienced enough to take good care of you?" Perhaps Dr. Gross was feeling insecure and wanted to get right into the medical pathology. Not surprising; it is hard enough to sort out the medical mysteries without worrying what your patient is thinking. But we are dealing with people, not bellies in distress, and we need to focus on the person with the illness as well as the illness. It doubles our trouble but it must be done.[9, 10]

Finally, we need to enlist the patient's cooperation. That seems a more important task when the patient is leaving our office or the hospital but needs doing even if we are about to send the patient up to the intensive care unit. To do that, we must explain a lot, offer alternatives, and reach agreement with the patient.

# CHIEF COMPLAINT

Dr. Vise: Well, Tom, how have you been feeling?

Mr. Thumb: Not so hot, Doctor. I ain't been feeling very good.

V: What sort of symptoms have you been having? Chest pain?

T: Yeah, I've had a little chest pain, not too bad, still some. Like I usually have. No real difference.

V: Has the pain been in the front? Center?

T: Sure, that's mostly where all right.

V: Taking the nitro pills? Do they help?

T: Not very much, no. Maybe a little.

V: All right. Are you still taking the same medicines as usual?

T: Except for the Lanoxin. You told me to change that.

V: OK. Well, let's take a look at you. How about taking off your shirt and sitting up here.

T: OK, Doc. The thing is, mostly I've just been feeling sick. I haven't been eating and I get these dry heaves in the morning.

V: Sick to your stomach?

T: Yeah.

V: Well, why didn't you tell me? Nausea and vomiting, eh? Any other stomach symptoms? Diarrhea? Are your bowels running?

T: No, they're OK.

V: OK. Well, hop up here on the examining table.

T: OK, Doc. What makes it hurt here in your stomach?

V: You're hurting in the belly?

T: Yeah.

V: Well, goodness. Any other problems you haven't told me of? Fevers?

T: No, no fever.

# DISCUSSION

Physicians who use questions as their main interview device waste a lot of time. Instead of asking the patient to tell his story and then getting out of his way, they are constantly putting themselves in the way of the story-telling. But one can do fairly well if he restricts most of his questions to large, open-ended ones such as "How have you been doing?", "How have you been feeling ill?", or "What sort of symptoms have you been having?" and avoids either closing off the potential answers or worse yet, indicating the sort of answer he wants.

This doctor was interested in symptoms and asked open questions but then abandoned them to focus on a single symptom. It seems that Dr. Vise cannot stand to leave an open-ended question alone. Immediately he narrows down the choices. "What sort of symptoms?" is immediately narrowed to "Chest pain?" "Belly symptoms?" is immediately narrowed to "Diarrhea?"

Worse yet, the symptom focused on was not the patient's choice, but that of the doctor. We'll never find out what is troubling our patient if we force him to address only our concerns and never ask what his are. Allowing this patient no time or space to choose his own area of concern keeps us from hearing his story.

By asking narrow-ended questions, this doctor never hears his patient's story. The result is that the patient is unfinished and keeps trying to go on. The doctor is soon going to be impatient and will probably blame his patient. "This fellow never gets to the point." Or "This fellow always has another symptom to tell you about. You never can finish with him." That should be no surprise. We usually blame our patients for our own flaws. This patient may remain unheard until the entire interaction is finished. Then, as the doctor has his hand on the doorknob, the patient will ask the familiar "By the way, doctor ..." question. If so, the cause may lie more with the doctor than the patient. If your patients are troubling you with "By the way doctor" questions, try a different interview technique. Before you are finished, list all their complaints and ask if there are any others you missed. Then wait for the answer. If the patient denies any others, ask again. "Anything else we missed or failed to cover?" And wait for the answer. Only then, should you go on.

By using a narrow questioning technique, this doctor maintains a high degree of control over the interview. He may think that he speeds things up in this manner, but paradoxically the patient's history takes longer. Thus, such an approach has several adverse results: the patient feels bullied and unheard, the process takes a long time, and the history may well be incomplete and misleading. It may be a surprise to learn that this is the very sort of approach many of our medical residents perfect during their residency training. They actually develop a more closed interview style as they progress through the training programs. My suspicion is that this technique is partly the result of spending many rotations on subspecialty services, on each of which the resident learns a long list of questions that elicit data pertinent to that subspecialty. At the end of several years of such training, the physician comes to believe that a good job of interviewing consists of asking all the questions asked by all the subspecialists. Of course, this is never possible in the time allotted. Instead, we must leave room through open questions for the patients to direct us to what's bothering them.

A most helpful interview tool turns out to be the chief complaint. Do we all agree on its definition? Mine is; 'the cardinal symptom as the patient views it'. It isn't the patient's biggest complaint. "Where is a fellow supposed to park around here?" won't do. Neither will "Your bill didn't come on time last month." Nor is it the patient's own self diagnosis: "I think my gall bladder is acting up again, Doc." Nor his idea of the correct therapy: "I thought I ought to come in for a shot of penicillin." It is a symptom, and it must be the most bothersome one to your patient, not to you.

How do you know which symptom? Ask the patient. "Of all these problems: chest pain, hip pain, dizziness, itchy rash, shortness of breath, and cough, which is the most bothersome to you?" When your patient shortens the list to three "I don't know, Doc, I guess the cough and the dizziness are worst. Them and the hip," you have to ask again. "OK, of those three: cough, dizziness, and hip pain, which is the absolute worst?" It may take a lot of doing to elicit the chief complaint. And obviously it may not be the first one the patient cites. It may pop up only well along into the conversation. But the chief complaint is still a very powerful tool. When you determine the cardinal symptom, that is the place to begin, even if you have spent a lot of time already.

Our formal history and physical examination forms often feature the chief complaint high up on the first page. That's a good idea. It leads the story and can help you best help your patient, but it may not be forthcoming early on in the interview. The final written transcript of the interview is not a verbatim record, but a construct, a narrative we create from the data we elicit. The chief complaint is what propels that narrative.

# WHERE WERE YOU YESTERDAY?

Mr. Hawk came to the office on Friday because of anterior chest pain and palpitations. He was known to have severe coronary artery disease, had been treated with a quadruple coronary artery bypass graft eight years before, and often had short runs of ventricular tachycardia. His regular doctor, Dr. Fred, was out of town until Monday. Mr. Hawk saw Dr. Fred's colleague, Dr. Lee, in the office and Dr. Lee admitted Mr. Hawk to the hospital's cardiac ward. He asked a cardiologist to see the patient in consultation. Dr. Roy, the cardiologist, had consulted for Mr. Hawk eight years ago and periodically since. Dr. Lee explained to Mr. Hawk that Dr. Fred would be back on Monday and that he, Dr. Lee, would also be gone over the weekend, but that Dr. Tim would be covering his and Dr. Fred's practice. Dr. Roy evaluated the patient and advised some changes of medications. He saw the patient on both weekend days as did Dr. Tim. On Monday, Dr. Fred returned and resumed care of his patient. Dr. Roy was out of town Monday, but had made arrangements for cardiac catheterization to be done on his return Tuesday. Tuesday morning, Dr. Fred was examining Mr. Hawk when Dr. Roy came in the room.

Dr. Rot: Hi, Joe, how are you feeling?

Mr. H: Where were you yesterday? My doctors are always off on vacation.

R: I wasn't on vacation; I was working. I had to go up to Santa Cruz and I did three caths. I worked my buns off.

H: Oh.

Dr. Roy then launched into a long, careful, detailed explanation of the cardiac catheterization to be performed that afternoon. The patient listened carefully. Then:

H: My heart's doing flip-flops again. I don't want that happening down in the heart lab.

R: That's OK. We can take care of those beats easily in the lab.

H: Unless you both are in Santa Cruz. If so, what then?

## DISCUSSION

Consider first the small dialogue that Dr. Roy thought was a joke on the part of his patient. "Where were you? My doctors are always on vacation" seemed a gentle bit of ribbing to him. The patient asked his question with a big smile on his face and Dr. Roy, used to having people clamor for his attention, thought it just a little joke.

We should be careful with the remarks we think are jokes by our patients. Often the humor veils a serious concern. If we assume that a patient is always asking about himself and about now, it isn't hard to imagine that this patient is asking whether his doctors will be available for him when he really needs them. He has just experienced a doctor run-around that would make your head spin. The physicians must look like a merry-go-round to him. Any one of them is likely to show up or not show up on a given day. Who is in charge? Who is responsible? Who will be there if he really needs them?

So how to answer his questions? One might try, "I can imagine that it is confusing and worrying to you when we seem to be out of town as often as in. You must wonder who will be there if you really need us."

Then, in that light, his concerns about palpitations and the upcoming cardiac study are easily placed. We need tell him not only that we can handle them during the catheterization study, but also that we will keep a close eye on him thereafter. We need to be specific about our availability. Of course, if we can just recognize his concern, we are likely to defuse his apprehension. We don't have to make promises we can't keep, just recognize his feelings and concerns.

# *HOW CAN I TRUST YOU?*

Ralph V. came to see his internist, said he was quite well, but asked that he be tested for HIV antibody. He denied any homosexual experiences or IV drug use and said that he had been happily married and monogamous for the last seven years, but he had been more promiscuous before his marriage and said that he would feel a lot better if he knew that he was HIV negative.

The physician, who cared for both Ralph and Ralph's wife, noted the lack of risk factors, explained the nature of the HIV test, and, somewhat reluctantly, ordered the test. One week later the test came back negative, as expected, and the doctor so informed his patient.

Three months later the physician received an irate call from Pamela V., Ralph's wife. She said that the couple was in marital therapy and that Ralph had just told her that he was bisexual and that he had had an extramarital love affair with another man during the early years of their marriage. "But," he reassured her, "I've had an HIV test at our doctor's office, and it was negative." Pamela was not as comforted as she was angered and called the doctor to say that she felt betrayed by his failure to tell her what he must have known about her husband. She felt betrayed by two men, her husband and her doctor. "How can I trust you?" she asked. "What other secrets are you keeping from me? How would I know?"

She was quite angry and the telephone steamed during the conversation. The doctor was flabbergasted by the news and felt unjustly accused.

## DISCUSSION

This is a rough one. There are two intellectual problems. The first is the fact that the doctor did not know what his patient is now surmising he knew. He didn't know about Ralph's bisexuality. The doctor must confess his ignorance. In a way, Ralph protected his doctor from the second and larger issue: how to deal with conflicting privacy issues and right-to-know issues.

Of course, the first difficulty is how to deal with anger. No one enjoys being the recipient of anger. If your ability to tolerate blame is low, being blamed by your patient may mobilize all your bad feelings and you might respond out of your own anger. Those responses escalate the problem. I find that it sometimes helps me to remind myself of just who is angry. This is an angry patient, one who feels hurt and mistreated. She may be misinformed, but she still feels exactly that way. Then it is fair, once she has finished saying what she had to say, to let her know what you heard.

"I can hear that you are angry and feel mistreated and betrayed by what you think happened here. If that were what happened, I would feel so too in your shoes. It might help some to know how things look from my point of view. Would you let me tell you?"

With that introduction, Pamela was willing to hear more and although still angry, she did listen. The doctor explained that he too had been lacking any information about Ralph's contacts and only knew that Ralph wanted the blood test done. New information like this can be a wrenching shock and many people are unable or unwilling to give up their posture of anger. But Pamela thought about it for a few seconds and then conceded that she couldn't expect her doctor to tell her what even he didn't know. Eventually she was able to forgive the doctor for what he hadn't done. Such flexibility and willingness to accept new information and act on it is rare. More often the angry person will not be able to give up his or her anger so quickly and we shouldn't expect them to. Pamela is a rare person who can both express her anger clearly and give it up when she decides it is unwarranted.

After the anger and hurt had been assuaged, the doctor needed another meeting to discuss the second, larger issue: how can a doctor handle conflicting needs of a married couple like this? I'm not sure what the optimal strategy is, but it seems that the more conversation about the issue, the better. I think the bulk of the conversation has to be with the first member of the partnership. The goal of that conversation would be to lead the patient to understand the dilemma that he and his doctor share. He must understand that the doctor can't carry some secrets with ease and is especially burdened if the failure to communicate could damage his second patient.

For the physician, it may be best to remember when you're doing a procedure where you anticipate that the results, even the doing of it, are to be of interest to other people, it is necessary to discuss these needs and to discuss them early on.

What if Ralph's blood test had been positive? In Colorado the HIV results are automatically reported to the Department of Health by the laboratory. And the doctor is legally obliged to report them. Then the Department of Health contacts the patient and attempts to trace contacts. This process has produced a great deal of controversy. Many claim that testing is hampered by a lack of anonymity. However we physicians in Colorado mostly applaud the public health efforts to keep careful track of this epidemic disease. And in an individual case the public health involvement solves our communication problems. We could say to Ralph, after he assimilated the initial shock, that Pamela was going to learn these results shortly via the public health department. Wouldn't it be better if she learned it from her husband and her doctor? And I suspect that a meeting of the three would be arranged quickly.

# WOULD YOU LIKE A BITE?

The patient, a 35-year old man, came to consult his mother's physician. He said that he was generally quite well but had become concerned about the swelling of his feet. He was a heavy smoker and drinker, smoking three packs of cigarettes a day and consuming two to three quarts of wine a day. Nonetheless he continued to run his business. He said that he assumed the alcohol was responsible for his leg swelling and he was willing to stop drinking. The physical examination was remarkably normal except for slight enlargement of the liver. He had no other stigmata of alcoholism and had no edema at the time of his initial examination. After a long discussion and some laboratory tests, the patient left the doctor's office promising to cease drinking immediately. He was begun on chlordiazepoxide and propranolol in moderate dosage and agreed to return in two days.

At the time of his return he was modestly tremulous and a bit anxious but mostly felt better. He had not drunk any more wine and he said that his family was very supportive. The biochemistry testing had been normal but for slight liver abnormalities. His albumin was 3.6 gm./dl. During the next three weeks he continued to feel better and better. The tranquilizer and propranolol were decreased and then discontinued. His liver function tests returned towards normal. However his edema worsened with each visit. Three weeks after he had stopped drinking he had four-plus edema of both legs, up to mid-thigh. No other abnormalities were evident.

Puzzled and worried, his doctor admitted Mr. S. to the hospital, planning to do abdominal CT scanning, venograms, and perhaps lymphangiograms. The doctor thought that some intra-abdominal vascular disaster was causing the edema, perhaps a thrombosis of the inferior vena cava or hepatic vein. He expected to have to begin the patient on intravenous heparin therapy at the very least. At admission, Dr. Fred arrived to re-examine his patient prior to the various tests. Mr. S. had just been admitted to his room and Mrs. S. was also present, looking for a place to sit.

The conversation went as follows:

Dr. F: Let's see, John, I want to check your blood pressure and then I want to go over you once again.

Mr. S: OK, Doc. Be my guest.

(Dr. F. busy with blood pressure apparatus.)

Mrs. S: (trying to manipulate the bed rail on the vacant bed in the room) How do you get the bed rail down? I can't seem to make it work.

Dr. F. (still busy) I'm sorry, that is a very important secret and we don't just tell it to anyone. There is a high price for such information.

Mrs. S: I don't know what to offer you. Would you like a piece of licorice? Can I offer you a bite of licorice?

Dr. F: Sure, I like licorice. Uh, Uh, Uh.


## DISCUSSION

Serendipity strikes again! Mrs. S. later said that she never before had actually seen a light bulb brighten over a person's head. I was the physician. It took a few seconds for the realization to work its way into my consciousness:

Dr. F: Licorice? Is John eating licorice? How much?

Mr. S's mother, a lovely woman, had been sympathetic to his distress recently and had been supplying him with her own version of panacea, 24-ounce bags of real licorice made with glycyrrhizic acid. I had last heard the licorice story about 20 years ago, and knew that it could cause pseudo-hyperaldosteronism with hypertension and hypo-kalemia, neither of which Mr. S. had. But it did seem possible that the licorice could be acting as a mineralocorticoid and could be responsible for the patient's edema, perhaps aided by his slight liver disfunction. All the x-ray studies were normal and the discontinuing of licorice cleared up the edema over the next two weeks.

I was amazed at this turn of events. If I hadn't been in a fey mood and indulged in a bit of teasing with Mrs. S., I would never have learned about the licorice. I would never have thought of asking about licorice. It was a miracle.

What is one to make of this conversational miracle? Surely it is the opposite of the usual conversational failures.

I don't know how to classify this sort of event. It seems clear that the doctor has to be there and has to allow room for the patient or his relative to speak, to say what seems unrelated to the matter at hand. There need be time, space, and permission. But that alone will not produce miraculous results. Sometimes this sort of event gives me the feeling that there are guardian angels for doctors. These close calls should increase our usual minimal humility. I missed this diagnosis entirely and only blundered to it by a most circuitous and surprising route.

We do well to preserve some humility and to be aware of the role of chance and accident in our diagnostic and therapeutic processes.

# BIG TALKER

Dr. Frame: Well, Mr. Gratt, what brings you in to see me today?

Mr. Gratt: My wife.

F: You are here because your wife suggested it?

G: Right.

F: Well then, what sort of trouble were you having that led her to suggest this visit?

G: You'll have to ask her.

F: And how are you feeling now?

G: Fine.

F: What did your wife notice that worried her?

G: Didn't ask her.

F: Hmmm. Did your wife accompany you here today?

G: Didn't bring her.

F: Well then, you came because your wife was disturbed, but you don't know what she was disturbed about and you are feeling fine.

G: Right.

F: A man of few words, I see.

G: Hmph.

F: Well, given all that, what would you like from me?

G: Dunno. You're the doctor.

F: OK. This is sort of "for you to know and me to find out, eh?"

G: ... (silence)

WHAT NOW?


## DISCUSSION

"What now?" depends on what you think is going on. Is this man holding out on Dr. Frame? Is he angry, perhaps, because he was obliged to come see the doctor? Does he have a perverted understanding of how doctors work so that he assumes things go best if he says the least? Is he remarkably inarticulate? Or is he confused, suffering from an organic brain syndrome?

If you think all these equally likely, you might do best to explain your problem to him. You might say, "Well, I'm having a lot of difficulty here. I need your help. I would like to help you if I can and to do so I need to understand what sort of symptoms you have been having, just how you have been feeling not-all-right. But we don't seem to be getting anywhere. Is there something getting in the way? For example, are you angry with me?"

The general technique of owning the trouble and then asking the patient for help in solving it has been called 'confrontation.' You can consider this technique as a confrontation of your problem, not of the problem patient. It does not imply any hostility. You do not, for example, shake your patient by the lapels and shout, "Look, you S.O.B., you better start cooperating or it's out on the streets with you." What you do is claim the difficulty and ask for help in resolving it. Such confrontational devices can include statements like "I am having trouble hearing you well, could you speak somewhat louder to me? I am a little bit hard of hearing." Or, "I notice that you seem to look away from me all the time. Are you angry with me or am I scaring you?" Perhaps a better term than 'confrontation' is 'enlistment in the engagement process.' To work together patient and doctor must be tightly engaged. I have an image of a railroad coupling device. The linkage has to be secure. If the linkage has come undone, we need to ask the patient's help, enlist him in re-engaging. I like that image better than that of confrontation.

In this case, confrontation or enlistment led nowhere. The patient denied fear or anger, seemed calm, but could not add anything to help. Dr. Frame next tried to evaluate the patient's memory and attention. He said "I wonder if you are having a little trouble remembering. How is your memory?"

No one wants to own up to being crazy or being demented but we all are willing to admit being a little forgetful now and then. I, for example, am willing to admit having "Sometimer's disease." This has been said to be an early form of Alzheimer's — you remember things sometimes.

Mr. Gratt admitted that his memory wasn't everything it had once been. That allowed the doctor to introduce a mental status examination. "Let me give you a little memory test. You don't have to worry about passing or failing it. I'm going to ask you about 30 questions. Just try to listen carefully to the questions and do the best you can." The mental status quiz he employed was particularly useful in diagnosing organicity.[12] Mr. Gratt scored 9 out of 30, an abysmal result. That clarified things to the point that Dr. Fuzzy ceased trying to get more historical data from a patient who could provide none.

# NO TRADITIONAL DOCTOR

Dr. Square: Hello, I'm Dr. S. Are you Ms. Flash?

Ms. F: Yes, doctor, I am.

Dr. S: What sort of troubles bring you to see me?

F: Before we start, doctor, I need to ask you a few questions to see if you are the right sort of doctor for me.

S: All right.

F: I was recommended to you by a friend of mine, Susan Splash. But I am concerned to know if you are the right sort of doctor for me. I am interested in finding a doctor who has some flexibility and isn't limited to traditional medicine.

S: What would that mean to you?

F: Well, I consult an acupuncturist and I buy my food from a health food store and I do regular Rolfing sessions and I want to be sure that my doctor understands those sorts of health measures.

S: Uh, huh. What other sorts of healthcare people do you consult?

F: Well, I have a chiropractor and sometimes I use a naturopathic psychotherapist. But it is important to me that my doctor be interested in holistic health and not just a traditional type.

S: I see. And what specific sort of medical problem have you been having lately?

F: Well, two years ago I developed a cancer of the breast. I had surgery and chemotherapy and the doctor I used to go to back home said I should be checked every year.

S: I see. Are you having any troubles now?

F: No, I have been feeling quite well. I think the high colonics I've been getting from my chiropractor have been helping. I want to make sure I do everything I can to avoid another experience like that one with the breast cancer.

S: You are indeed feeling fine?

F: Yes I am. I've been exercising a lot and my work is going well and I have been feeling well.

S: OK. What I think we should do is first review your past medical history, then do a physical examination, then talk about our findings.

We also will have to talk about the issue you brought up about the sort of physician I am. But let's start first with you.

F: OK, Doctor.

Supposing the history reveals no other significant medical issues and the physical examination is normal except for the missing left breast. You have told your new patient this good news. How are you now going to respond to her concern that you be a 'holistic' and non-traditional doctor? What to say?

## DISCUSSION

It seems to me that the doctor's goal is to be scrupulously honest with his patient, yet to avoid offending or insulting her. He must make an effort to clarify the epistomological framework he uses and yet try to remain available to her as a physician.

I would try something like this:

Dr. S:  About the traditional or non-traditional medicine question, I have some thoughts and would like to explain them to you. They may be different from your ideas though. I'm not even sure that we are close enough in our ideas to work together, but I hope we can and I will try.

I think there really is such a thing as traditional medicine. But I don't think you and I are referring to the same thing with that term. What I call traditional medicine has been around for many thousands of years. Practitioners of traditional medicine usually each have a favorite sort of treatment and they provide the same treatment for all their patients. One traditional practitioner may use manipulation for all ailments and another may use herbs, but there is likely to be little difference in treatment dependent on the patient's illness itself. There is a lot of faith involved. Rather than controlled studies to show that a specific treatment works, one just asks for belief in its efficacy.

Then, about 150 years ago a new approach was developed. It would be fair to call it scientific medicine. It is definitely not traditional. It depends on being able to demonstrate something in carefully controlled studies, in being able to achieve the same results in repeated trials, and in actions fitting with previously demonstrated knowledge of anatomy, physiology, and chemical interactions. Scientific medicine is young and very incomplete. Doctors who practice scientific medicine have to say "I don't know" a lot.

What I try to do is practice this sort of scientific medicine. So if you come to me for care, you will quite often hear me say that I don't know. I will promise to tell you what I do know and what I don't. That will often leave matters incomplete and you may find that you still want to consult some of your more traditional healers who always have a good answer and a treatment for everything. And I may have to say that I don't know if what they are doing might be helpful or not. About all I can really promise you is that I will stick with you, that I will try to hear you, and that I will be honest with you.

How does that sound?

This example is from a subset of the larger topic of how we share decision-making with our patients. If we try to address the physician dominance and the imbalance of power to empower our patients, we must share with our patients considerable information, even an understanding of our epistemology and our uncertainties.[13] In fact, patients who view their role as more active seem to do better under their doctor's care.[14, 15] This patient may turn out to be one of our favorites.

Finally, it might be that I am giving an example of my tendency to over-explain. Instead of a lecture, what this patient really needs is evidence that we understand her problem.

Dr. S  It sounds like you're caught in a dilemma. You want my help with scientific medicine and you're concerned that it may not fit with your other more traditional approaches. Perhaps you're concerned that I might ask you to give up an approach that you have confidence in. That would be a tough bind to be in.

# THE DISEASE YOUR DOCTOR
# DOESN'T KNOW

Ms. Qwerty: Hello, Doctor.

Dr. Brain: Hello. You must be Ms. Qwerty. I'm glad to know you.

Q: I've been going to Dr. Kwashiorkor for years, but we just changed our insurance and I had to switch doctors. Dr. Kwashiorkor suggested you.

B: I see. That must be distressing, having to leave a doctor you liked and trusted just because of an insurance change.

Q: It was, Doctor. And even more so since my problem is not one that most doctors understand. Are you familiar with the Yeast Disease? I brought some articles with me... (waving around a popular magazine with an article titled "The Disease Your Doctor Doesn't Know.")

B: The Yeast Disease?

Q: Yes, I have a yeast sensitivity. I do pretty well if I avoid anything that has yeast in it like beer or wine or fruits or carbohydrates and take my Nystatin and the vitamins and minerals but otherwise my life is miserable. Do you know anything about this disease? I know that very few doctors have ever studied any nutrition and that the AMA keeps this stuff hidden from you.

Do you? Do you know about the Yeast Disease?

## DISCUSSION

Are you filled with dread? Are you convinced that The Yeast Disease is a non-disease? Do you suspect that this patient will begin with no confidence in you and become still less trustful as matters proceed? Do you perhaps shudder when any patient begins with his or her diagnoses even if they are bonafide medical diagnoses? (One of my colleagues described a patient as "handing out diagnoses like credit cards.")

Irwin Press, a medical anthropologist at Notre Dame, says that every patient consulting a care-giver in any society comes with his own explanatory model (E.M.) and that we will never see a conscious patient without an E.M. If Press is right, we should assume that a patient has a diagnosis before consulting us. She has probably already consulted her family, friends, pharmacist, and others. Finding a name for something gives us the sense of having some control over it. No surprise that she comes to us with a diagnosis. And it is not brought as a punishment for us. In fact, with a little consideration, we can begin to look forward to the E.M. "Aha!" I say, "That is her explanatory model." Later on I can cite it to her: "You had this problem with your breathing (or whatever) and thought it might well be a yeast allergy acting up. That was a good idea, but I think it really is more a matter of..." Knowing and being able to give credit for the patient's diagnosis decreases her anxiety that she is not going to be heard. She may then be able to listen to your ideas. If you haven't heard her own diagnosis, you have no way to combat the patient's suspicion that you "didn't even consider that I have yeast disease." She will go away more satisfied if she understands that you gave consideration to her idea of what was going wrong.

Then, what to do with her questions about your knowledge and belief in this specific diagnosis and pathophysiologic analysis? How to avoid being queried about your belief in and knowledge about this non-disease?

Use the same technique we learned as medical students when a patient mentioned a disease we were not familiar with. Faced with a patient who says he has Osgood-Schlatter's Disease and is staring at him, the medical student learns to say: "Well, that disease affects different people in different ways. How is it affecting you?"

Dr. Brain: Yes, indeed I am familiar with it. However this disorder seems to affect different people in different ways. How is it affecting you? What sorts of symptoms does it cause?

If the patient remains unwilling to provide symptoms, you can explain your need and insist on the process. After all, it is your shop. You define the rules.

Dr. B: No, I really do need to understand your specific symptoms. Otherwise I'd be treating you just like everyone else with these sorts of disorders. And that would be no good. You are an individual and we must understand your symptoms.

Of course, the rub will come when you need to define future steps and therapy. What if your conclusions are that the patient has another problem? What if you want to treat the patient with something else than her usual Nystatin? This is especially hard for me. I often get my back up and become very inflexible at such points. But intellectually, I think you really do have to negotiate about these issues.[15] There really are disagreements between doctors and patients, disagreements about the nature of the problem, about the goals of therapy, and about the precise therapy to apply. And it is best not to discard her diagnosis, the one she is convinced of. Rather, you might add your own and suggest that we might do best to treat this other problem first while we gather some more data on her dietary symptoms, or whatever she describes. In fact, I think it is dangerous to completely discard any observations she has made, no matter how they fail to fit into standard pathophysiologic understanding. Sometime later you may even come to realize that she has been telling you about something new that you hadn't previously understood.

I remember the time a patient told me about his flatulent response to his ulcer regimen, a diet full of milk, right after I had read an article about lactase deficiency. I had surely heard similar stories from other patients before, but I had no framework to place the story on. Suddenly I knew what my patient was telling me about. Aha!, I thought, that's what all these people have been telling me, claiming an "allergy" to milk. Now I understand!

Perhaps someday an understanding will surface that will explain the Yeast Disease in a scientific framework. So we needn't deny the existence of such a problem, but can still do our own work with sense and integrity. On a good day, perhaps one in three, I can do that. Otherwise, I may get into a power struggle with the patient and our relationship disintegrates.

# A RASH IS A RASH

Dr. Rose: Hi, are you James Brooks? I'm Dr. Rose. I hear you are having some skin trouble.

B: Right. I have this silly rash on my leg. I've had it on and off for years. I usually come in and get a shot of Aristocort and it is fine for another year or so. That's what I came for today. I need a shot of Aristocort.

R: I don't understand. Your chart is very thin and I only see notes about you having a cold one or two times. When were you here about the rash?

B: Oh no, I wasn't here. That was the doctor I used to go to. He was in another clinic. I only need the shot of Aristocort when the rash flares up. I guess it's stress that brings it on.

R: How are you otherwise? Any other problems?

B: No, Doc, I'm fine. Look, I don't mean to be in such a rush but I got to get to a meeting in about an hour and it's clear across town.

R: OK. Let's have you strip down to just your shorts and put on this gown. I'll be right back and then I can get a look at your skin and see what we can do for it.

B: Look, Doc, it's not on my skin. Just here on my leg. I can pull up my pant leg and you can see all of it. I just need the shot of Aristocort and I'll get out of here.

R: I see. (The patient has pulled up his pant leg, exposing a small patch of red skin.) Still, I'm not sure that the Aristocort is the best therapy. Did your other doctor ever do a biopsy? I'd like to know the pathology.

B: Yeah, he did a biopsy. He said it was just dermatitis. He said there was no curing it and no use fussing with tests. He said just get a shot when it flares up and that's plenty. He was right. This is a waste of time.

R: I can imagine it must be very annoying to you to have this rash come back over and over.

B: (sounds angry) It's not that big a deal. It doesn't even pop out every year and a shot cures it each time. I don't know why we have to go through all this. A rash is a rash.

R: Well, would you mind if I just called your previous doctor and got the biopsy report first?

B: Sure that's OK. But I don't know how you'll find him. I don't even remember his name exactly and his clinic closed, I think.
Anyway, why don't you do that but in the mean time, if you'd give me that shot of Aristocort, I could get out of here.

R: Well, I suppose so. But just this once. Then we really need to do a complete exam and get that biopsy report.


## DISCUSSION

The central problem in this conversation is that of a patient who knows what therapy he wants and a doctor who doesn't want to be bullied.

This situation can easily produce a standoff. Sometimes the best approach is to name the difficulty. "We are having a real difference of opinion. You know from past experiences that a shot of Aristocort usually helps and you think that is the very thing to do now. I think that I haven't got a clear diagnosis yet and that I usually do better for my patients if I do have such a diagnosis. So how are we going to resolve this? Is there any way we can both feel satisfied?" Often, invited into the process of solving the interactional problem, the patient will join with the doctor and the problem easily solves itself. He may become much more helpful in other areas, too.

One line of this dialogue is especially interesting, the point when Dr. Rose allowed that it must be frustrating to have a recurring rash. This doctor had just come from a discussion of doctor-patient communication and was interested in the technique of empathy. She thought she would try such a technique and attempted to join with the patient by identifying what she thought was frustrating him: the recurrent behavior of his rash. That effort failed immediately. In fact, the patient became more angry and the doctor felt more annoyed at that point. But after the conversation was over, when asked what she thought was really aggravating her patient, she quickly answered, "He just wanted his shot of Aristocort and was angry that he wasn't getting it." If she had used that awareness to construct an empathic statement, she might have done better. She could have said to him, "It must be really annoying to you that you came here knowing exactly what sort of therapy would help and exactly what you wanted and here I am thinking of all sorts of reasons why we should do something else instead of what you want." Her patient would probably have agreed and have felt understood. The rapport generated by such an accurate empathic statement might not have solved their basic disagreement, but it would have helped narrow the distance between doctor and patient.

The key to empathy is that it includes a diagnostic guess. You must make a stab at describing what is paining your patient. As with other diagnoses, you may be wrong. But you are more likely to hit the target if you first think about it. Ask yourself, given what he has been saying, how he might be feeling. In this example the doctor really knew what her patient was unhappy about. She tried using empathy as a rote device instead of a piece of insight and it failed. No surprise.

# NURSING HOME CALL

Phone:  Ring, ring, ring, ring

Dr. Beetle:  (Dropping the phone, having just awakened at 11 PM)
Yeah? Hello?

Nurse Griffon:  This is Emily at Easter Health Center. Is Dr. Beetle
there?

B:  Yeah, this is me.

G:  Dr. Beetle, I am calling to confirm orders on your new patient,
Mr. Blair.  He was admitted on days but they didn't get his admission
orders confirmed.

B:  Who? Who is Blair?

G:  He was Dr. Anneberg's patient but Dr. Anneberg doesn't come to
Aurora Health so they assigned him to you. They said they had cleared
it with your office.

B:  Oh, OK. I suppose so. Well I've never seen him and don't know
him yet. Tell me about him.

G:  Well, he's on Keflex, Digoxin, Lasix, vitamin B12, thiamine ...

B:  Wait a minute. That won't help me until you tell me about him
first.  What's he like?

G:  Well, his diagnoses are atherosclerosis, degenerative joint
disease, congestive heart failure, BPH, and Alzheimer's disease.

B:  OK. That sounds like everyone else. What is he like? What do
you observe?

G:  Well, I haven't really seen him much. He seemed cheerful.

B:  Can he walk? Is he oriented? Tell me the vital signs and what
he looks like.

G:  I don't think he is walking now; he's asleep. He seemed to know
where he was and they said he ate his dinner. Let's see... his blood
pressure was 160/90 and I don't know if they got a temp.

B:  Emily, I'm not learning much. Don't you have some sort of
routine assessment sheet you use with new patients?

G:  Oh yes, Doctor. The day people do that. I didn't assess him
because he didn't come in on my shift. I'm just calling to get his orders
confirmed.

# DISCUSSION

Unfortunately these calls are becoming more common, perhaps the norm rather than the exception. It is a rare nursing home that has the administrative direction to require good data collection and good assessment of patients by it's staff. How many of the staff have any training in patient evaluation? Few nursing homes are willing to pay what it would take to carry such staff. Few use nurse practitioners or other trained patient examiners.

What can the doctor do?

One obvious challenge is to remain calm and avoid damaging your already flimsy working relationship with Nurse Griffon. She may not be very skilled or very diligent but she is likely to be quite sensitive to criticism. Nursing home staff tell many tales of angry doctors who shout at the nursing home staff on the phone. No surprise, but not much help either.

I've evolved a response that is not satisfactory but helps me feel a little less powerless. First I do point out my own vantage point, or more accurately, disadvantage point. I say that I am half asleep and would prefer being called during my usual day hours. Then I explain that I need to know all about the patient even to OK simple orders. I tell her to go back into the patient's room and look him over, wake him up and ascertain if he knows where he is and what day, month, year it is; to take fresh vital signs, look at his skin, see if he can stand and walk; then to call me back. I say that I will expect her call within 30 minutes. And I ask for the phone number of the director of nursing. Then, while she is examining her patient, I call the D.O.N., sometimes enjoying the thought of waking her, and explain my needs to be called during the day and for complete information when I am called. And I volunteer to come and give an inservice lecture on what staff should know before calling the doctor. Sometimes I am taken up on that. I explain that I depend on the director of nursing to solve these problems for me. I commiserate with her about the high turnover of nursing home staff and the low rate of pay that prevents them from hiring fully trained personnel. I ask her to not bother the staff that night because they are going about their work right now, as we speak, to gather the needed data.

Yes, the D.O.N. comments are really true. The turnover in nursing home staff is great. Most are paid little, come untrained and leave soon. Few nursing home administrators or nursing directors have any insight into the communication problem that develops when the patient becomes ill and a doctor must be called. This problem may be with us for a long time.

# THIS IS BUTCHERY

Your answering service called you at 11 PM Thursday night to tell you that a Susan Sverbota is calling about her mother, Annette Sverbota. You return the call.

Dr. Kindly: Hello, this is Dr. Kindly. Is there a Susan Sverbota there?

S: This is Susan Sverbota, Doctor. I was calling Dr. Gladly. Is he available?

K: No, Dr. Gladly isn't on call tonight. Can I help you?

S: Well, are you familiar with my mother's case?

K: No, I'm not. Tell me what the problem is.

S: I really wish I could talk with Dr. Gladly. He has been taking care of my mother for several weeks now and he knows all about her.

K: Well, he will be back tomorrow. Is it perhaps something that could wait till then?

S: No, I really want something done for my mother sooner. Are you sure Dr. Gladly can't be found?

K: Perhaps you ought tell me the problem.

S: Well my mother is in the Villa Vista Nursing Home and they are killing her. They are nothing but butchers there. They didn't give her the antibiotic Dr. Gladly ordered until I asked them why they hadn't given it. And they are starving her to death.

K: My goodness! That sounds terrible. How old is your mother? What sort of trouble does she have?

S: She's 95, Doctor. They think she has lung clots and heart disease. But that's no reason to starve her. Now she is unconscious and can't eat even if I try to help her. I think they ought to start an intravenous. You shouldn't have to die of starvation in America.

K: They aren't feeding her?

S: No. They said she didn't want to eat what they brought. But I know that she will eat if you cut the food up very small and if you sing to her when you feed her. Only now she won't take it from me either.

K: It sounds as if she is pretty sick, maybe dying.

S: That's what Dr. Gladly says. But I don't see why she has to die of starvation. You can die of cancer or big things but not of little things like this.

K: It is probably hard for you to see her like this. Hard to lose her.

S: That's not the point. She isn't getting good care. They left her all day and didn't make up her bed. They are evil people there. Butchers!

K: What would you like?

S: Well, maybe you could put her back in the hospital again and give her an intravenous. She might get better.

K: I think we should wait until morning. I'll talk with Dr. Gladly then. Would you like him to call you?

S: Can't we just start an intravenous now?

K: Let's just wait for morning. I'll talk with the nurse and then with Dr. Gladly.

S: All right, Doctor. Thank you.


You then call the nursing home and talk with the nurse on duty. She says that Mrs. Sverbota was just admitted two days ago. Dr. Gladly had said that she had terminal lung and heart failure and had been badly demented for several years. She was admitted for terminal care, with the expectation that she would die in a matter of days. She was to be made comfortable and such measures were being carried out.

The next day you talk with Dr. Gladly, who says that this patient had been in and out of hospital several times recently with no treatable disorders discovered. Her daughter had fired her previous doctor and the hospital administration had asked Dr. Gladly to take over her care. He had been spending an hour a day in conversation with the patient's daughter who seemed unable to accept the fact that her mother was dying. He says that he is tired of talking with her, will make one more effort and then will leave her to you since it is Friday and you are on call this weekend. He makes that phone call and you listen to his side of the conversation. It sounds as useless as yours did last night.

Saturday you receive another call from Susan Sverbota.

K: Hello, this is Dr. Kindly. Is this Ms. Sverbota?

S: Yes. Thank you for calling, Doctor. My mother isn't getting better. They aren't helping her. This is butchery. She needs an intravenous.

K: Would that really be helping her? Wouldn't that just be prolonging the dying process?

S: Well, maybe she'd get better. It isn't right to just let her die that way.

# DISCUSSION

This is a hard one. It may be too hard. Quite possibly the doctors who are identified as Ms. Sverbota's mother's doctors cannot be available to help Ms. S. who is clearly the person most in need of help. She will see such doctors as simple tools that she must use to get her plans accomplished. Someone else has to appear to help her.

The doctor might try a change of subject. He could say:

"I can see that we are at a bit of an impasse. We seem to have different ideas about what should be done for your mother. Could I stop for a minute and ask you a little about you? Could I ask how you are feeling in this situation when you are watching your mother dying and nothing you do seems to be helpful and you can't get any of the professionals you have found to help you as you would wish?"

Maybe, just maybe, she could leave the concern with her mother for a moment and tell you about her feelings instead of acting them out. But it is unlikely that the two of you could do such a therapeutic activity over the phone. And it may well be impossible for you to be helpful to her in any case since you are her mother's doctor, even in surrogate.

You might ask her if she has any other source of support right now, her own physician or a clergyman or a friend or a relative. Perhaps someone can be found who will be able to help her cope with the grief and anger she feels. Right now she is trapped with you and you are trapped with her.

As a matter of fact, after her mother died later in the next week, Ms. Sverbota tried desperately to get the city coroner to do an autopsy to prove that her mother had been murdered. Neither the coroner nor the hospital pathologists agreed to do such a study. At this point it is still unclear if anyone has been able to help Ms. Sverbota in her distress.

# NO BETTER, DOC

Dr. P: Hi, John, how are you feeling today?

J: No better, Doc. I just don't seem to get any better. I've been coughing just as much and I don't seem to be able to get to sleep.

P: Still trouble with the cough, eh? Is that what keeps you up at night?

J: I don't know, doc. Sometimes it seems that the cough just goes on and I don't get anything up. Then I just don't feel good. I'm sick and sometimes I get those fevers, too.

P: I see. Let's see now, last time I started you on an antibiotic.

J: Yeah. That didn't seem to help though. I took it a couple of times but it didn't make no difference so I quit.

P: A couple of times?

J: Yeah, I maybe took one or two a day for a couple of days.

P: Hmmm. What of the smoking? Are you still smoking?

J: Yeah, but I cut it down.

P: I see. How much are you smoking now?

J: Oh, I cut it down. I don't smoke more than about 15 or so cigarettes a day.

P: That's interesting. Last time you said you smoked about 3/4 of a pack a day. That sounds the same.

J: Yeah, but I used to smoke two packs a day. A couple of years ago I would go through more than a carton a week.

P: OK. Then what I hear is that you are no better than last week when I saw you. You are still coughing and still having fevers. But you are also still smoking and you've taken only a few capsules of the antibiotic I prescribed. Is that right?

J: Right, doc. I just ain't getting well. I've had this for weeks and I'm getting tired of feeling sick. When's this going to get better? Besides, I can't afford to keep coming here to see you if you can't get me well. I got to pay $10 each visit, on top of my insurance.

## DISCUSSION

This fellow isn't improving, isn't doing what his doctor suggests, and is beginning to be frustrated with what he considers to be inadequate doctoring. The doctor is feeling frustrated with inadequate patienting. What to do?

The doctor might try hammering at the same old song. He could rephrase, restate his suggestions. Maybe this time the patient will take his advice. Or he could try the lateral pitch ploy, referring the patient to someone else. "This seems to be a tougher problem than I thought. We ought to have you see a pulmonary specialist." Or he might see the problem as one of inadequate enlistment of the patient, in which case he would make efforts to enlist the patient in his own behalf.

Any such enlistment would probably take the form of some sort of confrontation, some effort to face the patient with his need to become the responsible agent for his own welfare. The doctor might just restate the problem: "It seems to me that this is very frustrating for you and even for me. You are not feeling any better, you are tired of feeling ill, and you are beginning to wonder just what sort of doctor you have who can let you stay sick so long. And I am beginning to wonder if there is any way I can encourage you to take responsibility for the health measures I think you need to get well. We are stuck here together." Then the doctor could clarify his perception. "From my point of view, you will not get well very fast unless you do at least two important things. One is to take the medicines that I prescribed and the other is to stop beating your lungs up with the cigarettes. How does that sound to you?"

That puts the ball in the patient's court. He may try to escape the responsibility: "Well, that cigarette stuff is old hat. Doctors have been telling me that for years. But this cough is a new problem. I've just had it a few weeks." The doctor can return the ball: "I can imagine how confusing it seems since you've been a smoker for a long time. But once you get an infection in the lungs, continuing to smoke keeps the lungs from clearing the infection. It's a lot like having a headache and pounding yourself on the head with a hammer. The hammering may not have been the initial cause of the headache, but it is hard for the headache to get better until you stop the hammering. What do you think you can do to improve your health now?"

What if your patient has another therapy to suggest? "My friend had a bad cold just like this and his doctor gave him a shot of penicillin and some vitamins and it was fine in a couple of days."

That's a little harder, but still best handled by admitting that you heard it, before explaining why it is not so good an idea. "I see. Your friend was ill, perhaps with the same sort of infection as you have, and after a shot of penicillin and some vitamins, got well. It seems logical to you that we do the same. Of course, I haven't examined your friend so I can't speak about his case, but for you, right now, with the specific sort of lung problem you have, it is quite unlikely that penicillin would be the best antibiotic. The antibiotic that has the best chance of helping you has to be given over a period of time, either intravenously several times a day, or by pill. And, if your lungs are unable to clear the infectious material because cigarette smoking stops the clearance mechanism, any amount of antibiotics will probably not help. So we are back to square one. What are you willing to do to try to help your own health?"

At some point, the doctor needs to stop arguing. This patient has all the information he needs. He must process it and take responsibility. The normal reaction to persuasion is to think of a counter-argument. Mark Twain described this problem in a short story [16] and Geoffrey Williams and colleagues recently modified Twain's argument to suggest a more therapeutic approach.[17] We might try silence:

P: Well I guess we're stuck.

J: What do you mean?

P: I think we won't go forward until you decide to do something.

J: What about that shot?

P: (silence)

J: No good, huh?

P: (nods silently)

J: I really got to decide about smoking, eh?

P: (nods silently)


It is sometimes necessary to put the patient in touch with the problem and leave him there. However Geoffrey Gordon and Larry Evans suggest a more kindly and helpful approach, emphasizing an empathic response to the patient's dilemma:

P: I can see that you are caught in a real dilemma.

J: What do you mean?

P: Well, you clearly want to get rid of your cough and I share that goal with you. But you also really enjoy the smoking and don't like the idea of quitting. It's hard to make healthy choices all the time.

J: Yeah, I guess that's true, Doc.

P: Well, then, what do you think you can do?

J: What do you mean? Aren't you going to give me something to fix my lungs?

P: Ah! I'd like to, if I could. But my job really is to fix what I can and to advise you about the rest. Your job is to work on whatever is keeping the infection and inflammation going, especially the smoking. What else is getting in the way of your doing that?

J: Oh, I tried to stop once.  Maybe I could again.

P: (nods, silently)

J: I'd like to stop.

P: It is really in your self interest.

J: OK, I'll do it. Can you help? I heard about those nicotine patches.

P: Right! Might help. Let me tell you about them.


However you choose to approach this patient, it is clear that persuasion isn't the optimal strategy and that knowledge is only the first step towards a behavior change.[18]

# POISONING

A 60-year-old woman was consulting her physician because of persisting headaches, dizziness, and malaise for the prior three weeks. The headaches involved her entire head and consisted of a dull ache, unassociated with visual symptoms, photophobia, nausea, or other neurologic symptoms. They tended to begin in the morning when she began her work as a salesperson at a large department store and often abated by afternoon. The general sense of dizziness and malaise seemed more pervasive. She had no other symptoms and the physical examination was entirely normal. A biochemical survey and CBC were normal and she was back in the office a week later to report no improvement in the symptoms and to hear about the normal blood tests.

Her doctor was puzzled.

Dr. Thoughtful: I am puzzled, Mrs. Lincoln. You seem quite troubled by all these symptoms but I can't find anything wrong. I am wondering about the possibility of some sort of an emotional cause. Are you, perhaps, depressed?

Mrs. Lincoln: Sure, I'm a little bit annoyed by being sick but I haven't felt particularly depressed lately. It's just that I don't feel well and have this headache and dizziness.

Dr. T: Well, I'm not sure what we ought to do next. Should we do a CAT scan or an MRI of your brain? I don't think it is very likely that we will learn anything. What other causes could there be for your symptoms? Is someone trying to poison you? Is your husband trying to cash in on your insurance?

L: (laughing) No, no, Doctor. He's a real sweetheart. He is so kind to me. I'm sure he's not poisoning me.

T: Well, sometimes these sorts of illnesses just take their time and go away by themselves without us really understanding them. Maybe that's what will happen here. Perhaps we should just wait a week or two and reconsider it if you are still not better.

L: OK, Doctor. I'll call you if anything is worse. Otherwise I'll come back in two weeks.

Two weeks later, Mrs. Lincoln returned.

T: I'm glad to see you. I've been a little concerned. How are you?

L: Oh, I'm fine now. I found out what was the trouble. My husband was poisoning me.

T: Now you're kidding me.

L: No, he really was. We figured it out. He's such a nice guy that every morning when he'd go out to the garage to leave for work, he'd start my car, too. Then when I'd come out in ten minutes or so, the car would be warm for my drive to work. But I kept the windows closed going to work, and by the time I got there I had a headache and was dizzy. I guess I hadn't realized that connection when I talked to you before. So I had Robert stop running my car and my troubles are all gone.

How did this solution appear? Another miracle? Is there anything the doctor can do to encourage the frequency of such solutions?

## DISCUSSION

Too simple to believe? Maybe. And, indeed, this case is not buttressed with any positive supporting laboratory data. By the time she was feeling better, the patient was not interested in re-doing the experiment just so her doctor could obtain a blood carboxy-hemoglobin level. And, of course, his diagnostic acumen hadn't been enough to lead him to that test when she was symptomatic. Nonetheless, I believe the diagnosis. For one thing, it was reached by the patient, not the doctor.

About the best I can say is that this doctor and his patient had so good a working relationship that he could suggest to her the possibility of poisoning without any really clear ideas of toxin or mechanism and the idea allowed her to think her own way to the right conclusion. In a way that is the ideal description of the doctor-patient relationship, a working partnership. Sometimes, perhaps usually, the doctor does the technical thinking. Sometimes the patient does. And when the patient comes up with an idea, it behooves the doctor to consider it seriously.

# ANY MEDICINES?

Dr. List: Are you taking any medicines?

Mr. Clean: No, just the Tagamet.

L: Tagamet? How often?

C: Just when I need it.

L: OK, how often is that?

C: Not too often.

L: Well, how many in a week.

C: Oh, hardly any. Maybe two or three times.

L: OK, what else? Any other pills or potions or medicines of any sort?

C: No, just the blood pressure medicine.

L: Oh yeah? What is that?

C: Tenormin. I take it once every day. I forget about it; it's just like a vitamin to me.

L: What do you mean, you "forget about it?"

C: Oh, I mean that I take it every day, but I forget to count it as a medicine.

L: Any others?

C: No. Just the breathing medicines for my asthma.

L: Uhuh. What is that?

C: That's when I get short-winded and can't hardly breathe. You remember, we did that breathing test once.

L: No, I meant what medicine are you using.

C: Well, not really any medicine. Just my whiffer. The thing I breathe in.

L: And which one is that? What's its name?

C: It's something like Probenyl. I use it just when I need it.

L: And how often does that turn out to be?

C: Oh there's no counting. Some weeks not at all and other weeks I use it ten times a day.

L: How about lately?

C: Oh, maybe two or three times a day. I take a couple of whiffs and I can breathe better without coughing so much.

L: OK. Let's see. We've got Tenormin and Proventil and Tagamet. Any others?

C: No Doc, except for the vitamins and the herb laxatives.

L: What vitamins?

C: I don't know exactly. My wife gets them down at the health food store. She gives them to me so I don't get cancer or prostate trouble. I think there's zinc and copper and B12, of course.

L: OK, anything else? Pain medicines? Headache pills? Water pills?

C: No, just some Extra Strength Excedrine. Just when I have a headache.

L: How often is that, I wonder.

C: Oh, not very often. Hardly any.

L: I still don't know how often that is.

C: I don't know, Doc. I just take them when I need them.

L: I wonder why we didn't have any of this written down in your chart.

C: I don't know, Doc. Nobody asked me that way. Anyway, I don't hardly take any medicines. I try to avoid them.


A conversation you never have?

Is there any danger in this sort of effort to clarify, with precision, the drug list?



# DISCUSSION

Of course you have this same conversation every day.

Part of the problem is the usual lack of precision in ordinary conversation. Most people are not in the habit of being precise about anything. Yet we need to know specifics. We need to know how long the symptom has been present, exactly when it appears, and exactly when it vanishes.

And when we insist on quantitative precision in our questions, including the task of recording symptoms or medicines, the conversation may seem controlling and intrusive to our patients. They may feel that they are the victims of a third degree inquisition. Sometimes we need to realize how oppressive our clarifying efforts can be. Our patient may, if we are lucky, tell us later that he or she felt overwhelmed by our apparent attack, by our querying approach.

Occasionally we meet the opposite problem, a patient who insists on over-precision, usually defining to a T the most innocuous phenomena and unimportant symptoms. The patient may want to list over-the-counter homeopathic remedies with intolerable specificity. What then? I think we have to resign ourselves to accepting precision, even when we don't much want it. After all, what is sauce for the goose is sauce for the gander.

# COMPLICARE WONT ALLOW

Ms. Strike: I'm sorry to bother you, Doctor, but your receptionist insisted that I come in. I really only need some referrals. I have to see my gynecologist and my ophthalmologist. You could have done that without my coming in and then you wouldn't have had to waste your time.

Dr. Form: I see. Let's see now, are you on some sort of insurance that insists that I refer you?

S: Yes, I have Complicare. You have to fill out a form.

F: I see. Well then, it would have saved you a trip in if I did this without seeing you, but not saved any time for me. Anyway, the problem is that Complicare insists that I see you first for non-emergent problems and they are very strict about when and whom we can send you to. They give us terrible grief if we don't follow their guidelines. Tell me about the problems you are having.

S: No problems, Doctor. That's why I didn't think I needed to come in.

F: I mean what is it that leads you to want to consult the ophthalmologist and the gynecologist.

S: Oh, just that it is time for my pap smear. My gynecologist says I have to come every year. And I haven't had my eyes checked for over a year.

F: Is your vision giving you trouble?

S: Oh no, it's fine. But Dr. Glassworks says I should come every year.

F: Uhuh. And I thought you had had a hysterectomy.

S: Yes that's right, I had everything taken out ten years ago. I had a fibroid and my periods were all messed up. Anyway I had had all the kids I needed. Things are better without periods.

F: Well, all that sounds fine. But I think I have some bad news for you. Complicare has pretty strict rules about use of subspecialists. They won't allow us to refer you if the problem is something that we ordinarily handle in our own office. That's why they call us primary care doctors. And we do routine pelvic exams all the time. We would usually only refer you to a gynecologist if there was a problem we couldn't handle or were puzzled by.

S: You mean you won't send me to Dr. Speculum?

F: Well, it is fine with me for you to consult whomever you wish. But Complicare won't allow us to refer you to him unless there is a problem beyond our expertise. You'd have to pay for your visit there if you went on your own.

S: That's preposterous! They made it quite clear that Dr. Speculum and Dr. Glassworks were on their referral list when I signed up.

F: True, but they also probably told you or wrote in all that insurance program gobbledegook that they sent you that all referrals depended on our OK and then they turned around and told us we were not allowed to send you unless the problem is outside our ability and our usual practice. I'm sorry and wish it were otherwise, but we are caught in the system much as you are. Anyway, how about if we go ahead and do the pelvic exam and see what the situation is. We probably wouldn't do a pap smear though because you have no uterus and the reason for a pap smear is to diagnose cancer of the cervix. You can't have that since you no longer have a cervix, I presume.

S: But Dr. Speculum told me I need a pap smear every year!

F: Uhuh. Well, let's take a look first and then talk about it.

S: I don't think I can do that today, Doctor. I will have to come back when I have more time. I don't want to do a pelvic exam today.

F: OK, we can schedule it in the future.

S: And what about Dr. Glassworks? He says I should have my eyes checked every year..

F: Oh me. That too. As I understand it, your vision is OK, right?

S: Right.

F: No eye pain, no trouble seeing or reading?

S: Well, sometimes I see little things floating by, little specks.

F: Uhuh. When I did the general exam last month, your eyes looked fine to me. And Complicare thinks that routine eye exams should be spaced out a little further in well people who are under 40 years old and have normal vision. They don't adhere to the ophthalmologists' requests for annual visits.

S: I don't believe it! This whole trip here wasted! I can't say that you are much help, Doctor. I never had this trouble when I used to go to Dr. Compliant.

## DISCUSSION

When asked about frustrating patient encounters, physicians today frequently cite the triangle involving insurance carrier or HMO, doctor, and patient. They say that they are increasingly being placed in an adversarial relation with their patient by insurance rules and regulations. They worry that "practice guidelines" will soon exacerbate the difficulty.

How to deal with this frustrating bit of news for the patient without alienating her and destroying any hope of working together? Whatever is done, it is likely to take a fair amount of time. This is another example of a matter that seems of little medical importance taking a great deal of time. Just as the time spent educating a patient about an illness is inversely proportionate to the severity of the illness, so the time that must be spent discussing administrative matters will always be much more than either patient or doctor wanted it to be.

Secondly, there is no harm in trying to empathize with the patient. It may not work miracles; your patient may still be angry. But it is reasonable to say that you can understand how annoyed she must be with you and with the new system she's found herself in. "I can imagine that this experience is very aggravating for you. I could understand if you are angry with me." Are you tempted to add: "But we both really know that I didn't design this system trap that we both have fallen in?" I am. However, excusing yourself and joining with the patient as co-victim of the system is probably not so very therapeutic. Maybe later, when passion has died down, you can point that out.

Perhaps she will point it out to you.

# MY PHARMACIST SAYS

Dr. Charles:  Good morning! I'm glad to see you, John; how have things been going?

John:  Not so good, Doctor. I've still got that pain.

C:  I'm sorry to hear that. Have you been taking the ranitidine?

J:  Well, not really. My pharmacist said that I had to watch out, taking it with Dilantin. So I just take one now and then.

C:  I see. And you say the pain is still in your stomach?

J:  Yeah, some in my back too.

C:  What do you think of that?

J:  Well, my chiropractor says that it is a bad alignment and that he needs to get my back lined up. He's been working on it. So far though, I still hurt.

C:  I see. Are you taking any other medicines?

J:  Just some Valium that I got from my sister. She thinks it's mostly my nerves. I've been under a lot of stress at work.

C:  Uh huh. So your sister is prescribing Valium, your chiropractor is doing manipulation, and your pharmacist warned you away from the ranitidine. Are you getting any other medical advice? I mean other than here?

J:  Not really. Some of my friends at the office tell me what they think and of course my mother is always poking vitamins and calcium down me, but otherwise, I don't have any other doctors. But the pain has really been worse lately and I've been taking more of the bicarbonate.


# DISCUSSION

Vaughn Keller, designer of the Miles Workshop on doctor-patient communication, likes to point out that people do not live in a dyadic relationship with their physician. Usually we can depend on our patients to have discussed their problems with family, friends, coworkers, and allied health workers, even some we may consider less-than-allied. Our patients come with ideas about diagnosis and ideas about therapy.

Initially it may seem annoying to discover that your patient is not following your recommendations but rather following those of every Tom, Dick, and Harry he meets. But you might reconsider. First of all, your recommendations carry a heavier weight and valance with the patient. Your patient may be hesitant to follow your instructions because of his perception of the power of your therapies. Judging other sources of advice as less potentially dangerous, he follows them. Well, that is almost a compliment.

Secondly, his telling you all this gives you an entry to discuss the problem and gives you invaluable information. Without this little saga of obtaining-medical-advice, you would know much less about your patient's style of dealing with illness and doctors. You would be puzzled about his failure to improve.

Probably the universal approach to this sort of problem is to share your difficulty with your patient. You could say: "I'm having some difficulty understanding this. It seems that you accept and act on all sorts of medical advice, except for that you have paid for from me. It seems that your care gets fragmented and falls apart when you do everything everyone says and I am not surprised that my therapy doesn't work very well if you don't take it. What could I do to help you with all this?" You might ask what he would like of you. You can gently point out that your therapy usually works better if he takes it as you recommend than it does if he doesn't. You might tell him that you do appreciate his telling you about other recommendations he's had, since that lets you understand better what he did and why.

Somehow you need to reach a better agreement about what the patient is going to do. Patient adherence to therapy has been shown to improve when the patient perceives you as concerned with his well being. Surely getting angry with him or blaming him for his divergence from your plans will not lead him to see you as caring or concerned. Before he leaves, though, you and he must come to some sort of agreement.

You might try reminding your patient that he really has two problems: the illness and the therapy. You can offer to help with both. Then, the problem you face is to enlist his full energy to cooperate with your plan and maybe to alter the plan to better fit his capabilities and his willingness.

You can say that you know what you advised him to do but you want to know what he actually thinks he will be able to do. "Will you be able to take this medicine twice a day? If not, how often do you think you would be able to take it?" He is much more likely to carry out a therapy that he has committed himself to.

# *HUH?*

Dr. G: Hello, I'm Dr. Graf. Are you David Crockett?

D: Yeah.

G: I'm glad to know you. The chart says you are 27 years old. Tell me a little about yourself.

D: Huh?

G: Well, for example, what do you do?

D: Ya mean work?

G: Yes.

D: Factory work.

G: Yes? What exactly do you do?

D: I do assembly.

G: Uhuh. And what do you assemble?

D: Huh?

G: What do you work on?

D: Da assembly line. Window shades.

G: And are you married? Single?

D: Single.

G: OK. How is your health.

D: Huh? Good, I guess.

G: OK. Then what brings you to me today?

D: I uhnknow. Sick, I guess.

G: In what way?

D: Huh?

G: In what way are you sick?

D: Uhnknow. Just sick.

G: Can you tell me more about the symptoms you are having?

D: Huh?

G: Symptoms? How exactly are you feeling not well? Pains? Short of breath? Fevers? Sick to your stomach?

D: Yeah, just, like that, sick.

## DISCUSSION

Not very articulate, eh? Maybe you are considering the D word (dumb). There are plenty of people out there whose vocabularies can be counted on your fingers and toes. If he were with his buddies, his conversation would perhaps be full of the F word. He might be one of those who can say an entire paragraph with nothing but the F word used in all its intonations.

Unfortunately, being inarticulate is not the same as being insensitive and, of course, he is quite able to be ill. You still have to establish some sort of relationship with him, try to sort out his illness, and establish a plan that he will be able to adhere to.

What about the technical terms of more than one syllable that he is able to use? "Assembly," for example. No surprise. Inarticulate people can often use quite long words. It is the task of fashioning new sentences with new thoughts that is difficult.

I wouldn't give up yet on the history. You may need to explain your needs very carefully and then ask your questions in a more narrow form, just the opposite from what we usually recommend. You might explain: "I will try to help you with this illness you have. To do that, it helps if I can understand the symptoms you have been having and then examine you. Then I have to try to figure out just what sort of illness this is and then just what treatment would be best for it. So to start with, let's go back to symptoms. Are you having pain?" Then you might list, one at a time, the common symptoms: itch, nausea, vomiting, diarrhea, shortness of breath, cough, chilling, fatigue, and so on.

# MY LAST DOCTOR MESSED ME UP

John Henry: Hello, Doctor. Mary Lewis suggested that I come to you. She says you are a very good doctor.

Dr. Yarnell: That's very nice of her. What sort of trouble are you having?

JH: Well, the main problem is that my last doctor messed me up.

Y: Oh? How was that?

JH: He didn't give me the right medicines and then he got me more sick than I was before.

Y: And how are you sick now?

JH: Just the same as I've been all along. Except that I'm worse since he messed me up.

## DISCUSSION

There are a lot of patient agendas that do not match with ours. We need to recognize that we are faced with one when it appears. Unless there is an emergent need that supercedes it, you then probably ought to attend to the patient agenda and to its non-congruence with your role.

Dr. Y: Uhuh. I hear you saying that your last doctor messed you up. I gather this is an important concern of yours. Perhaps you can tell me some more about that.

In fact, this patient's agenda may give you some pain. You may feel torn between supporting your colleague or supporting the patient. You can empathize with the patient: "That must have been distressing for you," perhaps offer to help patch up the communication problem, ask what the patient would like, ask for a promise of a discussion with you if you and he have a future falling out. You probably ought to beware of feeling proud for being this patient's new doctor or assuming you would never have "messed him up." Patients sometimes employ splitting, playing good doctor, bad doctor. Your exalted state may be only temporary.

Dr. Geoffrey Gordon suggests that we be specially wary of a patient who approaches us with "I want you to prove just how the other doctor messed me up." or "He wouldn't give me disability but I know you will." That latter might be specific to Dr. Gordon's work in a VA hospital.

And, if the patient wants to talk on and on about this, you might have to explain the time constraints.

Y: Well, I can see that I ought to hear you fully on this subject. But then to help you medically, I probably need to hear the story of your illness fully, too. Then I will need to spend time examining you and finally spend time thinking about the whole matter. We can't do all that today. What would be best for you? We could shelve the matter of your previous care until your next visit here. Or we could make you another appointment in the next few days to deal with your medical problem. What would you like to do?

# MY CHIROPRACTOR SAYS

R.J.R.: I don't want to take up much of your time today, Doctor. My chiropractor says that I need Dilaudid, so I came by for a prescription.

Dr. A: Hmm. Well, what I usually do is listen to the story of the illness and examine you and then come to some sort of conclusion about diagnosis and therapy. I don't think I can just be a prescribing arm of your chiropractor. Would you like to tell me about your trouble?

R: Well, the biggest trouble is that I have so much pain. My chiropractor says my back is so badly aligned that even he may not be able to get it into shape. I've been working on it with him for the last month. He says you'll need to give me a hefty dose of dilaudid just to get me up and working a little.

A: Tell me about the pain.

R: Not much to tell, Doctor. It just hurts. It's been hurting since I was injured so badly at work. They made me push a stamping machine at work and I strained my back. I heard it give way. My chiropractor says there is a lot of misalignment now. He says they ought to put me on disability. Anyway, I need more pain relief than I'm getting now. Last week I could hardly bowl without the pain stopping me.

A: Where is the pain?

R: In my back. I said I injured my back. When my chiropractor pulls on it, I hear it snap back, but that doesn't last and I hurt again when I get home.

A: OK, as I understand it, you have been having back pain just since you pushed the stamping machine, you have been getting therapy from your chiropractor, and now you want me to prescribe a class I narcotic for you.

R: Hey, I don't know nothing about classes of narcotics. I just want to get rid of this pain. I've had lots of back pain in my life, but those guys at work sure messed me up now.

## DISCUSSION

This story is enough to send shivers up and down the spine of most doctors. "My favorite confluence of difficult problems," says one. "An outside authority, especially one whose scientific validity I doubt. Then clear cut drug seeking behavior on the part of the patient, and strong hints of compensation problems, too. I feel trapped even before I begin."

No one obliges us to enter traps when we see them. If you were a bear and you recognized a bear trap, would you just put your foot in it? "Oh, this is a bear trap, I think I'll just put my foot in it." No self respecting bear would do it. Neither should you.

You might think that your therapeutic possibilities will grow if you accede to the patient's wishes this time and then form a therapeutic alliance and work in your preferred direction more in the future. Maybe. But maybe not. If you do accede, you might make it clear how much you are willing to do and how much not. My preference is to stop early. You have already spent some time with the patient and you are aware that things are not going the way you think they must go. Why throw good time after bad?

You really have a decision to make. Mine might be to tell this patient that he's come to the wrong fellow and that I can't help him; no charge for the visit, of course, but I'm not the person for him. A better decision might be to do some empathic limit setting. Then you could offer a real, if unlikely, route of working together.

You might say:

"OK. I have to say some things that you probably won't like. What I'm going to say might make you angry or unhappy. But I don't feel that I can give you that prescription. In fact, I am afraid that we may be in the wrong place, you and I. It might be that I will not be able to help you. I am under real constraints and cannot just fill the prescription of another healthcare worker. If I am to try to help you, I have to treat you just like any other patient. I have to take a full history, do a good examination, and come to my own conclusions. And they may well not include narcotic pain medicines. I know that this isn't what you came for. Perhaps you won't want to work with me at all. But if you do, it will have to be the way I described. I'd like to know your thoughts on this. Also I need to know if you thought there were any other things we could do for you besides the narcotic prescription."

# DID THAT MAN NEED HOSPITALIZATION?

(Thanks to Dr. Robert Berris)

You are in the midst of a busy office schedule when your assistant, Margaret, interrupts to tell you that you have an emergency call.

Dr. Berris: Hello, this is Dr. Berris.

Ms. Swat: Hello, Doctor, this is Estelle Swat. I'm a quality assurance reviewer for National Health Insurance. I need some information about your patient, William Wan.

B: Wan? He's in the hospital.

S: Yes, Dr. Berris, and your office did not notify us prior to admission so we are obliged to talk directly to the doctor to be sure of utilization criteria.

B: What do you need to know?

S: Well, first off, what outpatient care did you give prior to hospitalization?

B: What do you mean? I've been caring for this fellow for five years. You want to know all of that?

S: Oh no, Doctor, just the last two weeks. What did you do and what might you have done to prevent the need for this hospitalization?

B: I don't know what you mean. He was pretty sick. Fever of 104, wasting away, looked really sick.

S: Yes, but did you do any outpatient testing? After all, what we most need to know is did that man need hospitalization?

B: Look, he came in at 4:30 pm and looked terribly sick. I thought he needed to be in the hospital.

S: Well, we consider outpatient care to include the common infectious disease entities.

B: Do you come to take care of them? Look, he's got AIDS and diarrhea and cough and a high fever and has lost 15 pounds in the last two months and the guy is dying if we don't do something fast.

S:  Well, all right, Doctor you needn't get upset. I'll put down "gradual decline, not responding to outpatient measures." We can give you three days for that.

B:  What then? Send him home?

S:  No, no, Doctor. That just means that I or another reviewer will call you again at the end of the week. And don't forget, we will be glad to assist your hospital discharge planner if she just calls our 800 number.

B:  So I get to talk with you again on Friday?

S:  Probably not me, Doctor, I'll be off. But yes, one of our reviewers will check with you. Have a nice day!

B:  You've fixed that!

B:  Margaret, if that woman ever calls again, tell her I have migrated to New Zealand.

# DISCUSSION

A sign of the times. More and more time spent (wasted?) talking with third party payers. Do you suspect them of harassment? Maybe so. An editorial in the *Wall Street Journal* on January 2, 1987 described HMO disincentives aimed at discouraging physician involvement. Maybe other insurance carriers have found the same strategy. Dr. William Anderson suggested that disincentives to the health care providers would make them marginally less interested in serving the patients of that program. Maybe so.

On the other hand, insurance company utilization reviewers often try to get adequate, simple information from doctors' office staffs, information as simple as admission diagnoses, and find that no one knows what is going on. Then, of course, the reviewers have a hard time getting past phone barriers to get to the physician. In such situations the insurance companies often rely on the ploy of hiring physicians in practice to call and get the information doctor to doctor.

What strategy have you evolved to deal with these calls? Is it in any way related to the strategy you use to deal with dinner time phone salespeople who are purveying aluminum siding? Do you put them on interminable hold? Do you tell them long stories about your uncle Willie? Do you ask them to wait a moment so you can get a cup of coffee, take off your shoes, relax and enjoy the conversation? Do you tell them they have no business describing their call as an emergency? Do you ask the caller for her home number so you can call her at her

dinner time? Or at midnight? Are you simply polite, brief, and suc-
cinct? If the latter, does it leave you with a dark bitter taste that dis-
quiets you through the rest of your day?

This is a situation for which I have no constructive suggestions. I
think we need some creative and inventive approaches. So far, mine
are fairly dull and not altogether satisfactory. I try to remember that
this person is trying to do her job and didn't design the procedure. But I
do say that I am very busy and would appreciate her brevity. I do ask
for her full name and write it down and use it during the conversation. I believe that anonymity leads to shabbier performances. And if,
in the end, I am convinced that my assistant could have provided the
information just as well as I, I say so and ask her to please try harder
next time to get all possible information from my assistant before
asking for me. Perhaps because my assistants usually try to do a thorough job, I find I am handling fewer and fewer such calls.

# WELL, FRED, IT'S LIKE THIS

The new patient, Dennis Becker, is 30 years old. His chart identifies him as an advertising agent. He is a husky young man wearing a suit and tie.

Dr. P: Hello, are you Dennis Becker? I'm Fred Platt. I'm glad to know you.

DB: I'm glad to know you too, Fred. I was sent here by Phil Yarnell. He said you might be able to help me.

P: Um hmm.

DB: Do you mind if I call you Fred?

P: Well, hmm. I suppose my natural inclination would be to call you Mr. Becker until we were better acquainted and I guess I'd be a little more comfortable at first if you called me Doctor Platt. Of course lots of my patients do call me Fred and that is my name.

DB: Oh, well, I'm sorry. I didn't want to offend you.

P: That's OK. I'm not offended.

DB: Well, then, I have been having this awful pain in my stomach.

P: Can you tell me about it?

DB: Well, Fred, it's like this. I've been hurting in the pit of my stomach. It wakes me up at night and comes on anytime at all. I'm afraid I might have pancreatitis or maybe a cancer like that actor.

P: Does the pain go anywhere else?

DB: Not really. Just that it really hurts a lot.

P: What other symptoms are you having?

DB: Well, Fred, sometimes I get this awful burning under my breastbone. I get it sometimes after sex.

## DISCUSSION

In fact, I am a little uncomfortable with some patients calling me by my first name, especially if they are new to the office. So several questions appear.

Why didn't I admit to that discomfort? Why not be straight about it? Do I want the ease of my own informality (witness my introducing myself by name rather than as Dr. Platt) and still hope to keep the patient in a more formal structure? Maybe I need to go back to introducing myself as Dr. Platt, if I want to be called that by the patient.

I do remember observing an older physician 20 years ago who introduced himself to a patient in the emergency room as Stuart Smith. I admired Dr. Smith and thought I'd follow that manner. Now I wonder how Dr. Smith liked his patients to address him.

Second, why is this patient intent on using first names? Does he find that more comfortable? Perhaps it's a style he uses in his work? Or is it some sort of subtle put-down. If so, why? Is he overwhelmed by the usual, anxiety and dread, and trying to reduce the dread by treating the dreaded object, the doctor, with less respect?

Third, now that we are in this situation, now that I have allowed the uncomfortable first name conversation to go on, what should I do to remedy it?

A colleague suggests that I tell my patient that I'd prefer he not use my first name until we have him feeling better. "When you're cured will be the right time for that." Such a suggestion is whimsical enough for me. I might do that. But I probably also have to explain that I wasn't really aware of my discomfort at first, that Mr. Becker probably sensed something I hadn't yet realized, and that I would indeed prefer for us to be more formal at first. Then I could add the plan for holding first names until my patient is cured of whatever it is. I could then ask him how all that sounded to him, whether it was much ado about nothing, and whether he could cope with that request from me.

After I thought awhile about this matter, I did call Dr. Smith, who has now left his surgical practice and works part-time in an outpatient clinic. I asked him how he came to introduce himself as Stuart Smith instead of Dr. Smith. He told me that he was fortunate to be the student of some fine physicians who taught him about politeness when he was quite young. Then, prior to his surgical residency, he worked as a small town physician caring for a population that he viewed as "very competent people." He cared for ranchers and farmers and thought of himself as a consultant and a colleague to them. It made more sense to him to introduce himself to them by name than as Dr. Smith. Of course, he admitted, they already knew he was the doctor. Finally, he told me that he thinks our greatest task in medicine lies in increasing patient responsibility. He thinks we do that best by decreasing the hierarchical distance between us and them. As I heard his comments, I thought that perhaps I would continue to introduce myself as Fred Platt and that, if my patient wanted to call me Fred, I would try to be happy with that result.

However, I've asked other colleagues about this sort of problem. Dr. Herbert Kennison told me that it was his least favorite patient syndrome. But then he explained that he did nothing and said nothing to the patient about it. Why not? He told me "I don't like it but I'd rather not mention my discomfort." That brings up another issue, our tendency to swallow up our own distresses. Sometimes we do that long enough that we finally erupt in anger, usually discharging the patient from our care. I don't think we should allow our distress to build up so. We'd never advise a patient to do it. So, if it is painful, I think we ought to talk about it with the patient, hard as that is.

# I DON'T HAVE TIME
# FOR BEING SICK

Mr. Great: Hello, Doctor, how have you been?

Dr. Lopez: Pretty good, Winston, how about you?

G: Well, I've been all right, except for that gall bladder problem.

L: How has it been bothering you?

G: Just the same, Doctor. I get those bouts of pain in my right upper quadrant. They don't seem qualitatively any different and you know that you did that ultrasound and found out that I have a cluster of stones. You said stones and gravel, as I recall. The bother is that the attacks seem to be more frequent. And last week I had one that lasted four hours and I couldn't accomplish anything at work. I almost went home.

L: Ah. How frequent are they now?

G: I had three last week. Two were the usual half hour events and the one long one. One of the shorter pains woke me up and I walked around for half an hour. The other was during a lunch meeting and I just kept going. Before that they were more like once a week.

L: I see. Even once a week is more frequent than you had told me when I saw you four months ago. I see in my chart notes that you were then having them every two or three weeks and by the way, I had thought I'd see you before now.

G: That's right, Doctor, I missed an appointment. I had an emergency board meeting.

L: That's all right. What have you decided you want to do about the gall bladder? As I recall, we talked about lithotripsy, chemotherapy, laparoscopic surgery, and standard surgery.

G: Well, I read the material you gave me and don't think I want lithotripsy or drugs. And I'm a little unsure about the laparoscopic surgery since it is so new and might end up having more complications. So I guess I favor standard surgery, but the truth is I just don't have time for it.

L: You don't have time for it?

G: Right. I don't have time to be sick and I don't have time for an operation. My schedule is booked solid for the next six months.

L:  Well, Winston, it sounds as if you need to consult a surgeon to have an opinion about the matter anyway. Can we get you to discuss the matter with a good gall bladder surgeon?

G:  I really don't have time right now, Doctor. I'll just have to put it off until next spring.

L:  Hmm. You might not have as much control over this as you'd like. If you have another attack it might last even longer and then you might need emergency surgery. Recovery from emergency surgery can take longer than it does after an elective operation. If we're dealing with an attack of acute cholecystitis, the illness is much worse than simple biliary colic. We've talked about this a couple of times, I think.

G:  Well that might be, but I just can't afford to be sick right now. There is no way I can fit it in.

## DISCUSSION

Unfortunately, the patient's sense of time availability won't interest his gall bladder. Gall bladders are like the weather — they don't care what we think. So he may have to make room, like it or not.

Dr. Bill Lopez says this case is about denial. He's probably correct. But we have a schizoid view of our patients' attitudes towards illness. When they are hopeful beyond their expectations but their hopes do not conflict with our plans, we extol their style and say that they have hope and that it is a good thing. When their views of reality offer hope beyond what we deem likely and these hopes lead to behavior that conflicts with our plans, we call it denial. I think denial is the other side of hope.

Besides, I like to consider this case to be about hubris. I like this Greek term for pride. We suffer from hubris when we believe that we can control for our fate. We deny the capricious nature of the forces that have our lives in their hands. I don't know who the god of gall bladders was, but he has his eye on Mr. Great and Mr. Great is now about to learn that he cannot schedule his illnesses as he can his administrative meetings.

Hubris isn't limited to our patients. Physicians surely suffer from pride. It is our occupational hazard. In fact, by pointing out this sort of patient pride, we may fall into it ourselves, thinking that our awareness of reality is a step above the ordinary. I have to watch out for the sin of pride as I gently tell my patients that their ordinary life concerns must now take second place when they enter my sphere. Although there is no sign over my door proclaiming "Abandon Hope All Ye

Who Enter Here," sometimes I operate as if there were a sign saying "Abandon All Your Ordinary Concerns, All Ye Who Enter Here."

What should we do with this patient? After all, the future course he takes is his own choice. He can elect to wait until his disease gets him into enough trouble that he cannot disregard it. We don't have to abandon him just because he doesn't want to do as we suggest. I think our main obligation is to set the options out for him quite clearly and then agree to stand by and to stick with him, whatever he decides. But if he is operating under excessive denial, it might be worthwhile to face him with it. We have to make a real effort to enlist him in his own care. I'd try this:

L: Winston, let me see if I understand. You know that your gall bladder is a sort of keg of explosives that might explode any time. You take trips frequently and the explosion might happen when you are away from home, with uncertain medical care, unfamiliar doctors, and an unknown surgeon. You would like to deny the existence of your biliary disease and just pretend that it isn't there, but it won't go away whatever amount of attention you give it.

What a dilemma! On one hand you could die of a ruptured, infected gall bladder. On the other hand, you have to lose business opportunities if you take time off to have the gall bladder removed. How are you going to make the decision?

Then I'd be very quiet and let him stew with the problem. I wouldn't change the subject or accept any other turn of the conversation for several minutes. Maybe, just maybe, he would give it his focused attention.Whatever he chooses, we should write the choice down in his medical record, including the pros and cons of the choices as we've discussed them. We can ask whom else he has consulted and ask for other data that gets in the way of deciding for our recommended option. And we can clearly point out the hazards of each choice and ask him if that is really what he wants to happen.

# THERE'S ONLY ONE HALF,
# AND THAT'S MINE!

Sitting at a nursing station at the hospital, we can overhear half a telephone conversation between a staff cardiologist and the wife of his patient.

Dr. Ronald:  Mrs. Bill? This is Dr. Ronald at St. Righthere. You can send someone to pick up your husband.  I can't keep him in the hospital any longer. He's got to go home.

...

Dr. R:  Well, he still has a fever and we haven't been able to find a cause. But he has to go home. I can't keep him in the hospital.

...

Dr. R:  Yes, well, send someone for him. Then you have to watch his temperature and call Dr. Smith or Dr. Jones if he gets a high fever. I just can't fight with him any more. He insists on going home.

When asked about the case, after his phone call was finished, Dr. Ronald explained that two weeks after his coronary artery bypass grafting, Mr. Bill was still having daily fevers. Dr. Ronald thought that the cause of the fevers was probably a benign and self-limiting process such as atelectasis or the post-pericardiotomy syndrome, but he was still worried and would have preferred to keep the patient in this tertiary care hospital. Instead, at the patient's insistence, he was being discharged to his home in a small city 200 miles away, where there was a hospital but one less well equipped and staffed.

About his own feelings, Dr. Ronald said: "I hate having to go in to see patients and do two things, doctoring and persuading." When told that the new term for "persuading" was "enlisting the patient in his own care," Dr. Ronald replied that "those terms are all just bullshit. They all mean the same." Later, when I asked if I could visit with his patient to hear the other half of the story, Dr. Ronald thought such a visit not to be a good idea and vehemently replied: "There isn't another half. There's only one half and that's mine!" I thought that he said this last with a twinkle in his eye, and perhaps an awareness of his own exaggeration, but I could not help wondering if he really felt that way.

What do you think?

## DISCUSSION

One has to suspect that Dr. Ronald is a doctor of the old school. Perhaps he favors telling the patient what to do and having the patient respond, "Yes, doctor." Wouldn't we all! Unfortunately, most studies of patient adherence or compliance show that patients don't just do what we wish, even if they do respond "yes, doctor." In fact, adherence to our recommendations is often about 50%. So we need a new approach beyond telling the patient just what he is to do.

That better approach is some form of negotiation.[15,19] And, to give Dr. R his due, he probably did negotiate some future plan with Mr. Bill. Such a negotiation might sound like this:

Dr. H: Well, Mr. Bill, we seem to be at a standoff. I think you should stay here in the hospital and you think you should go home.

B: That's right, Doc. I'm going. I've been here too long and there's no two ways about it. I'm going.

R: OK, I can understand. Well, if you insist on going home, let's talk about what you would be willing to do that I think might be helpful to your health.

B: Like what?

R: First, I think we need to know what your temperature does. Can you take it twice a day and write the numbers down and let your doctors at home know how it is doing?

B: Sure, Doc. That's easy. My wife will like to do that.

R: OK, the second part is harder. If you get another high temperature you may need to be back in the hospital, perhaps the one at home.

B: I know that, Doc. I just can't stand to stay here any longer. I'd be willing to check in with Dr. Smith at home.

R: Fine. You know that I am still concerned about your fever and don't want anything to go wrong after you've been brave enough to go through with such an important operation.

B: I know, Doc, and I don't blame you for wanting me to stay here. But I can't stand it anymore.

R:  OK. Finally, can I get you to call my office in a week to tell me how things are doing?

B:  Sure. You know, if you let me out, none of those things seems too hard to do.


With such a negotiation, we may quickly realize that this patient will accede to almost any requests other than the one big one, that he stay put in our hospital. And the doctor and the patient end on a better note, in agreement and going the same direction.

What of Dr. Ronald's belief that doctoring is a different job than persuading? I have a hard time understanding that belief. We care for people, not circulatory systems. And we need the person to assume responsibility for most of his own care, for cessation of smoking, for dietary manipulations, and for taking medications. Only an anesthetized patient gives up responsibility. During the CABG operation we have to take over all responsibility, but before and after we have to educate and enlist our patients. That is all part of doctoring and I see no way to push the challenges of education and enlistment away and still be a doctor. We can be technicians without efforts to enlist our patients but we cannot be doctors.

This physician is known to be a very cautious, thorough, diligent worker. He is careful and attentive to his professional tasks. Since he takes his work very seriously, it may be hard for him to cope with a patient who seems headed in a direction opposite to what Dr. Ronald recommends. And Dr. Ronald has had a long career in a highly esteemed medical subspecialty. He has experienced a lot of patients who appeared to listen avidly to his every word and he may be convinced that they then did whatever he suggested. Many of his patients are quite vulnerable, frightened, and dependent when he cares for them. They are more likely, in that state, to accede to his wishes. But it is hard to imagine that they have always remained so cooperative when they achieved any independence, especially when they left the hospital. I doubt that even Dr. Ronald could be fooling himself to that extent.

Several days after this interaction, I reminded Dr. Ronald of his wonderful line, "There's only one half and that's mine." He became angry and insisted that he had never said any such thing, that I had imagined it. Perhaps so, but I wrote the line down the moment I heard it and I know that we are all capable of saying things we didn't realize we said. My conclusion now is that Dr. Ronald no longer believes he said that, but that he does believe that there is only one half to the story and that is his half.

# YES, DOCTOR, BUT

Mrs. Spratt: Doctor, you've got to help me. I absolutely need to take some weight off. I can't even fit into the clothes I bought last spring. This is the heaviest I've ever been.

Dr. Prang: OK. Do you have any idea what you're eating now?

S: Oh, I hardly eat at all. I often don't have anything for breakfast or at most, half a grapefruit and one piece of unbuttered whole grain toast and a cup of black coffee.

P: And the rest of the day?

S: Oh, hardly anything. For lunch I usually have a small cottage cheese salad and two rye crisps. And maybe a diet Pepsi.

P: And then?

S: Well, I usually have a normal meal in the evening. Then I am sometimes so hungry that I just keep eating all evening until I go to bed.

P: Like what?

S: Oh, I don't keep track, just whatever is around.

P: It might help to keep track.

S: I suppose so, doctor, but I can't imagine it's all that much.

P: What about exercise?

S: That's a good idea, doctor. Would running help me lose weight?

P: Sure it would. I wonder if just fast walking wouldn't be better for you at first.

S: Yes, but I have trouble with my feet, remember. I have those bunions and they hurt when I walk much.

P: Well there are other forms of aerobic exercise — a stationary bicycle, for example.

S: Yes, but they are so expensive aren't they?

P: Perhaps. There are usually some available for less than $100. though and you might find a good used bike by watching the want ads. Of course, none of these strategies is much good if you don't use it.

S: Yes, I thought of that, but I don't know when I'd find the time to do that much exercising.

P: You know, I think that your primary focus should be on what you eat, if you really want to lose weight.

S: Oh yes, Doctor, I do. But I don't think I can go to any of those fat programs. I tried Weight Watchers once and it didn't help.

P: You might begin by keeping a careful record of exactly what you eat and then trying to convert it into calories with a good calorie-counting book. I'd be willing to help you with that.

S: Oh that sounds like a good idea. But, I tried it once and I couldn't ever seem to remember to write down everything.

Have you ever had one of these conversations? What's going on? Any escape?

## DISCUSSION

Eric Berne described this routine in *Games People Play*. He called the game "Why don't you? Yes, but."

Some people like to play this game but I would not recommend it. For the primary player it leads to inevitable failure at whatever that person is trying to accomplish. For the secondary player, the role this doctor is assuming, it leads to immense frustration.

I think that the physician has to recognize the routine and label it as such.

P: Ms. Spratt, what we are doing right now is playing a hand of 'Yes, but.' That will get us nowhere. In fact, I don't much like to play that game and I think I am going to quit.

S: But Doctor, what will I do then? I can't go on being fat.

P: Oh no, I'm not going to do it anymore.

S: Do what?

P: Give you suggestions that you can use to explain why they won't work.

S: Well, what then?

P: What do you want?

S: I want to lose weight.

P: Uh huh. And what are you going to do to accomplish that goal?

S: Well, I don't know. Maybe I ought to keep a record of what I eat.

P: That might be a good first step.

S: But just keeping a record won't get me slender.

P: (silence)

S: Doctor?

P: Yes?

S: Just keeping a record won't get me slender.

P: (silence)

S: Of course, maybe if I see what I'm eating, I can try to change it.

P: That might be.


As you might imagine, some of my colleagues believe that silence does serve as a powerful device to get the ball back to this patient and to allow her to take charge of her fate, but that it may be too brutal a device to use. These colleagues recommend a gentler way to teach her to pick up the ball and take charge. They recommend an empathic restatement of the bind she finds herself in:

P: You're really in a bind, aren't you, Ms. Spratt?

S: What do you mean?

P: You want desperately to lose weight but any step you can see seems too hard for you.

S: I guess so.

P: Do you see anything you could do?

S: I'm not sure.

P: I can see that. You really are caught in a dilemma.

S: I might be able to keep a record of what I eat.

P: Uh huh.

S: And maybe if I see what I'm eating, I could try to change it.

P: I like that idea.

# WHAT WAS THE QUESTION?

Mrs. Pall: You told me to come back if I have more pain and I've been having a lot of trouble in my right arm. It hurts a lot. It just keeps me from doing anything.

Dr. Khan: I see. Exactly where does it hurt?

P: It doesn't hurt all the time. Sometimes it doesn't hurt at all. I don't know when it's going to act up.

K: I see. Tell me where it hurts the most.

P: Some days not at all. Yesterday was bad though. I couldn't even do any gardening.

K: Mrs. Pall, where does it hurt you?

P: In my arm, in the right arm. (moving her arm around vigorously, to demonstrate.)

K: And where in the arm is it most painful?

P: My husband says it's probably just arthritis and I will have to live with it.

K: OK, what else is bothering you?

P: Just that same old pain in my intestines. I think it's just gas. (rubbing her low abdomen, right to left, vigorously.)

K: And besides the arm pain and the belly pain? Anything else?

P: Just that swelling in my left elbow, except that it's fine now. Should I ask the orthopedist about my arm too? I don't feel bad today but you said I should come back in if my intestines act up again, so here I am.

## DISCUSSION

Does the patient's failure to answer a simple question such as "Where does it hurt?" drive you to distraction? What do you think the problem is? Did you not ask clearly enough? Do you not have her attention? Does she have a personality disorder? A thinking disorder? Has she never learned to listen to what other people say or ask?

It seems quite common, whatever the cause, that people don't answer simple questions, instead going on in their own direction. We can, perhaps, gain by listening to the direction they go. But if we need answers to our questions, we need to obtain those answers and I think that we often need to tell our patients that they have to listen to our questions and answer them.

I suspect that some people have never developed much conversational skill and tend not to listen to themselves or to others. We are often at fault in just that fashion, so it behooves us to be patient with our patients when they show the same flaws. But we need to get the critical information. It isn't much help just to blame the patient:

K: For heaven's sake, Mrs. Paul, will you ever stop your talk and listen to my questions?

P: You've no call to talk to me that way, Doctor, I'm just trying to explain to you.

Better to try to own the difficulty and ask for help:

K: Mrs. Paul, I'm having some difficulty and I really need your help. If I am to help you, I need to understand your pain very clearly. First of all I need you to listen very carefully to my question.

P: What question?

K: OK, here it is. Can you tell me exactly where in your arm the pain is most intense?

P: I told you, some days it doesn't hurt at all, I have to do things and I can. Today it's OK.

K: No, no. Please, Mrs. Paul. I need you to listen. I am not asking when it hurts, but where. Show me the most painful spot in your arm. When it hurts, where is that?

P: Oh, right here. (Pointing to the upper anterior third of the right upper arm.)

K: OK, great! That helps a lot.

Maybe this patient isn't so unfocussed in her account. She may just have a radically different view of what her story consists of. Elliot Mishler in *The Discourse of Medicine*[K], describes two entirely different, and conflicting voices, the voice of the life world, and the voice of medicine. We are used to the latter but use the former in describing our own travails throughout life. The patient has available only the former but is obliged to try to satisfy us by answering our queries with statements in the medical voice. In this case the patient is more concerned with "when" than with "where" the pain occurs. No wonder, "when" seems to her to help explain the even more important question, "why?" As doctors, we need to hear both voices, her story that has great concern for causation and responsibility, and our sort of story that answers questions such as "where it hurts?", "how long it hurts?" and so on.

# BY THE WAY

The patient had come to the doctor with a sprained ankle. The interview and examination were complete. The physician had recommended and placed an elastic bandage and was leaving the room, hand on the doorknob, when the patient said:

Mr. Rice: By the way, Doctor, what do you do when someone vomits up black stuff?

Dr. A: What do you mean? Have you done that?

R: Well, only a couple of times. Last week I ran in practice and then I vomited and it was all black. Then I felt OK again. And it happened a couple of weeks ago.

A: Why didn't you mention that before?

R: I guess I forgot. Probably it's not important.

A: No, that isn't it. I just thought we were finished. OK, tell me more about it. Any belly pain? Any other symptoms?

## DISCUSSION

Under time demands, feeling rushed and behind as most office practitioners are, the "By the way" or "Say, doctor" question strikes dread in the heartiest practitioner.

Thinking himself finished with that patient, almost out of the room, the doctor discovers that the most important problem hadn't even been broached.

How to avoid it? Perhaps no solution will work all the time, but the incidence of this disaster can be cut to a fraction by simply asking, earlier in the interview, "What else is bothering you?" And I suggest a rule of three: anything worth asking is worth asking three times. So ask "What else?" If nothing comes forth, ask again, "Besides the ankle problem, is there anything else you want to discuss today?" And, if still no yield, try a third time before comforting yourself that you have fully mined that vein. "OK, you have the trouble with your ankle. Is there anything more?"

These sorts of questions, asked as soon as you think you have defined the present illness, also serve as an emptying device for the review of systems. Are you troubled by patients who have positive reviews of systems, answering "yes" to your every query? If you precede the ROS by reviewing what you have heard about the patient's difficulty and asking for other current active problems, there should be little left in the ROS that is either important, active, or current. "Besides the ankle trouble, are you having any other current active problems?"

Stimulated by the Miles workshops on physician-patient communication that was developed by Vaughn Keller and Greg Carroll, I have tried to include several new questions in my every interview. They include "What else is troubling you?", "Is there anything else you wanted to accomplish here today?", "What did you think the trouble was? What sort of an explanation had you arrived at?", and "Do you have any questions we haven't answered yet?" I find that these five queries lead to easier interactions and I can get out of the room when I think I am finished.

Of course, once we elicit all the concerns, the list may be long. We needn't feel obligated to deal with all of them today. We can prioritize and deal only with the top two or three.

# WHY ARE YOU HERE?

The patient was a 40-year-old woman who came to consult the doctor about some bruises she had sustained when she bumped her head on a kitchen cabinet four days before. She had then stumbled and scraped her elbow and knee.

The doctor examined his patient and found nothing abnormal — no noticeable bruises, scrapes, or other abnormalities.

Dr. A: You look fine to me.

B: OK, Doctor, I just thought I ought to check.

A: OK.

B: Well I suppose I should have a Pap smear in six months or so.

A: That would be fine.

The doctor sat and thought for a moment. He realized that he had no idea why the patient was there. Her injuries were too trivial and too old to account for the visit.

A: You know, Barbara, I really don't exactly know why you came in today. Is there something else going on?

B: No, not really. Except for stresses at home, of course.

A: Like what?

B: Well, my husband lost his job. And he doesn't do nothing but sit around all day. He won't help out at home and he doesn't help with the kids. He brings his friends over and they sit and drink beer and make a mess and he expects me to clean it up. Then I have to come home from work and make dinner. I got so mad the other day when I came home and everything was a mess and nothing had been even started for dinner that I was rushing around cleaning up and I slipped and hit my head.

A: Sounds really frustrating.

B: You aren't kidding. I get so mad at him that I even hit him. He doesn't hit back but I really get angry. And sometimes I am awfully angry with the kids too. I don't hit them but I shout at them and then they cry. I just don't seem able to cope anymore. My nerves are just shot.

A: That is really hard on you.

B: I wish he would do something. Help with the house or go out and get a job or make dinner or something. I have to do everything and I just can't. Sometimes I'm afraid that I'll kill him, I get so mad. Do you think I could have some Valium or something for my nerves?

A: Maybe that would help, but I'd also like to hear more about the situation first and more about your feelings. Do you have anyone to help out at all? Have you talked with your husband about all this? Would it help for both of you to come in and talk with me?

# DISCUSSION

This is an alert doctor. He caught on to the fact that he didn't know why his patient was consulting him, even before the patient left the office. The realization that I am lost usually comes to me several hours later, much after the patient goes home. Then I have to call her back up on the phone and ask the critical questions. Much better to come to that realization earlier, while the patient is still there. Barsky described several "hidden reasons" that patients visit doctors.[20] I think it is best to ask the patient. We can follow Molde and Baker's recommendations [21] to search out the "iatrotropic stimulus" with questions like "How did you hope I could help you today?" and "Is there anything else you wanted to accomplish today?" Those two seem helpful to me.

Finally, when we are puzzled, we can take a little time out to think. In the BBC dramatization of John La Carre's *Tinker, Tailor, Soldier, Spy*, Alec Guiness, as Smiley, asked "What's going on here, John, what's going on?" I liked that question and the posture it portrayed. I thought it demonstrated the best medical posture, one of puzzlement and thoughtfulness. I also like the four-picture frontispiece from Cushing's biography of Osler. The photos show Osler looking, listening, palpating, and finally thinking. We might consider thinking more. It is not outlawed in medicine, although it is not done as frequently as it might be. We can even tell our patients that we are going to do it and ask their indulgence:

"Excuse me for a minute, Barbara, I have to think about what you've said."

That would surprise them, wouldn't it?

# I'M SO TIRED

Dr. Wise: Well, Sharon, what sort of trouble have you been having? What brings you to see me?

S: Doctor, I don't know what the trouble is. I'm so tired. I'm just tired all the time.

W: Do you mean you are weak?

S: No, just fatigued. I start the day tired and I stay tired. I go to bed tired and I wake up tired. I think I must have that EB virus thing.

W: Uh huh. Any other symptoms? Pain? Anything else?

S: No, Doctor, I'd be fine if I ever had any energy.

W: I see. How are you sleeping?

S: I don't sleep very well. I fall asleep OK but then I toss and turn all night. I wake up tired and I go to bed tired. Do you think I have that new disease? That EB Virus thing?

## DISCUSSION

As if the chief complaint of fatigue weren't difficult enough, now all our patients bring the diagnosis of EB virus antibody disease, a dubious diagnosis at best. But the symptom of fatigue is bona fide and quite common. I think the best description I've read of the chronic fatigue syndrome is Kleinman's chapter, "Neurasthenia: Weakness and Exhaustion in the United States and China."[0] Nothing else I know of so well clarifies the ubiquity and timelessness of this syndrome.

Chronic fatigue is probably the most common symptom that patients bring to us, yet we seem largely baffled by it and frustrated with such patients. Many authors view chronic fatigue as most often a mood disorder, usually depression.[22] I also find the following three mechanisms to be common in functional fatigue, i.e. fatigue that is day long, that may lighten a bit as the day progresses, that may be improved by exercise, and is not accompanied by signs or symptoms of organ failure, infection, or malignancy.

1. SLEEP DEPRIVATION. Carefully inquire about sleep patterns. If the sleep is disrupted by noise, light, depression, or unresolved conflict, the end result is sleep deprivation and pervasive fatigue.

2. A major UNRESOLVED DECISION. Debating whether to leave the spouse, the job, the home, the boyfriend, whatever, can lead to chronic fatigue as its main physical symptom.

3. LACK OF EXERCISE. Paradoxically, fatigue that seems to be the result of "working too hard" or of too much exercise, can be the result of too little. The best diagnostic test is a vigorous exercise program. I view exercise as a vitamin that is essential to good health; its absence produces chronic fatigue.

There is a 'chronic fatigue syndrome' that has recently been defined that has features of an ongoing immunologic or infectious disorder but that probably numbers far fewer than 5% of the patients who present with chronic fatigue. It is this syndrome that may have elevated antibodies to the EB virus.

About the patient's own diagnosis, "that EB virus thing," it is usually necessary to hear the patient's ideas and say that you've heard them. Then go on from there. Usually you don't need to deliver a long lecture about EB virus antibody titers and the new disease, 'yuppie flu'.

W: I know you thought EB virus disease might be causing your trouble, but I suspect it has more to do with the sleep deprivation we've noted.

S: OK, Doctor, I just wondered.

# WHILE WE'RE HERE

The doctor had just finished ministering to Mrs. Waller's needs. She has chronic rheumatoid arthritis and is being treated with low dose prednisone, organic gold injections, and aspirin.

Dr. How: All right, Mrs. Waller, I will ask Carla to get some blood from you to check your white cells and then to give you a shot of the Solganol. I'd like to see you again in a month unless you are having troubles. If you have any new problems, call us and come in earlier.

Mrs. W: Fine, Doctor. I'm really doing much better since you started that new medicine.

Mr. Waller: Before you go, Doctor, would you look at this wart I have on my thumb? I thought that while we're here you could just burn it off.

Dr. H: Yes, I see that you do have a nice wart. How long have you had it?

Mr. W: Oh it's been there for years. I've got a lot of back pain lately too.

H: Back pain?

W: Yeah. I get it every year or so and the last week has been rough. Since I changed the tire on my truck last week, I've been stiff and sore. While we're here, why don't you give me a prescription for it? Last time my old doctor gave me a muscle relaxant and it did the trick.

H: What else?

W: Oh I get some heartburn, but I take some Tums and it's OK. I'm fine. I just thought we could get it all done at the same time.

## DISCUSSION

Want to chew him out? Feel diminished by Mr. Waller's lack of appreciation for your valuable time? Wish he would schedule his visits like everyone else?

Or are you tempted to try to do what he says?

I suppose that it might be a quiet day for you and you might take on Mr. Waller's problems. But if not, there is no reason not to explain your needs. If you treat him with respect, you can expect him to treat you similarly. And if you treat yourself with respect, you might find that he will do the same.

H: Mr. Waller, it probably sounds simple to you and you must think that I could just do those two things for you. But to me it looks a little more complicated. To do you justice I need more time than I have right now, and the best I can offer is to see you in the next few days if you will make an appointment. I need to have enough time to focus on you and on your needs and not do a sloppy job of it. It would be unfair to my other patients whom I've promised my time and it would be bad medicine to you if I tried to rush you through and do a second rate job on you right now. I need to review your history and do a good back exam if I am to tend to your sore back, and that takes some time. And even the wart takes more time than I have just now. I don't want you to feel uncared for, but I really need you to come back when we have the time to do you justice.

What if you are one of the doctors who work in situations where they cannot schedule the patient back in a timely fashion? There are physicians who attempt to practice primary care medicine but whose schedules prevent them from ever seeing their patients when the patients are newly sick. All their ill patients have to appear at walk-in clinics or an emergency room. I don't know how to solve such a problem but at the least, the doctor should try to make an arrangement for Mr. W. to be seen somewhere, soon, by some medical person.

# ACUTE MYELOCYTIC LEUKEMIA

Dr. Perch: Hello, Mr. Longway, I'm Dr. Perch. I need to talk with you and then do an examination. Mrs. Longway, do you want to stay or would you like to leave us?

Mrs. L: I think I should stay. Could I?

P: Sure, maybe you will want to go out during the examination. (Turns to Mr. L) I'll sit here next to your bed. How are you doing this morning?

L: Weaker.

P: OK. And what brings you into the hospital?

L: Weakness. That and vomiting. And my white corpuscles, my blood count is down.

P: Tell me more about how you were before. Were you nauseated or did you just vomit?

L: Both. Nauseated and vomited both.

P: OK. Let's go back to the beginning.

L: How far back?

P: As far back as you think.

Mrs. L: He's been sick since March.

L: Well, I guess that first I ought to say that I think this was a shallow way of detecting disease. You go to the doctor with what you think is an infection on your chest. He gives you pills and you take them for a couple of weeks and don't get no better so you come back and he gives you a shot of penicillin. Then he starts thinking and gets an X-ray and it goes to Hayes, Kansas to be looked at. Then the next trip in you end up in the hospital.

P: When did you say that all began?

L: About April.

Mrs. L: He really wasn't well back in February.

P: Where are you from?

L: I ran out of gas. I live in St. Francis, Kansas. We're ranchers. At least that's what we used to be.

Mrs. L: He kept complaining of being tired. Then Dr. Cram gave him a big shot. We have a trilevel house and he likes showers but he couldn't do the stairs.

P: How long was it from "running out of gas" to not being able to climb stairs?

Mrs. L: It was acute. Only one or two weeks.

P: OK. And what did the doctor do then?

L: He did tests. He looked into my oxygen and found no oxygen in the blood. Then he did a bone marrow.

P: What did that show?

L: Acute myelocytic leukemia.

P: OK, so then he transferred you here? How have you been feeling since then?

L: Great. Until it gets time to be turned loose. We went home and I don't know if the doctor didn't explain it right or we didn't understand right.

Mrs. L: I didn't get the doctor's instructions right. Dr. Marrow, the oncologist, wanted us to check his temperature every day and I misunderstood him.

P: So why did you come here this time?

L: We tried to call Dr. Marrow and he was away. Dr. Cram was gone, too, to see the eclipse in Hawaii. That doesn't mean anything though.

P: How were you sick at that time, just before you came in?

L: I was weak.

Mrs. L: And that yeast infection had landed in his knee.

P: Any other problems with infections? Coughing? Any sputum?

Mrs. L: Oh he had a cough all right. The sputum was so stringy that he couldn't cough it up and I'd have to pull it out of his mouth. He was too weak.

P: Anything else? You said you vomited. Ever vomited blood?

L: Yes.

P: Any lumps or swellings?

L: No.


What does "OK" mean? Where might an empathic response be used in this conversation?

# DISCUSSION

There is a lot to discuss in this interview. But most important is to note that the patient, the patient's wife, and the doctor seemed to get along well. At the end of the examination the patient thanked his doctor and expressed desire to see him again in the future. I think that the doctor expressed a gentle caring and an acceptance of both the patient and the patient's wife that left them feeling better. That is our goal, for the patient to feel better when we are done.

However we should pay attention to two features of this doctor's technique. First is the interesting use of the word "OK." What do we mean by OK? What does this doctor mean?

Much of the time "OK" carries the same message as "good" or at least "acceptable." It is not equivalent to "Oh, how awful!" or "I am sorry to hear that news." But this doctor, when asked what he meant by "OK," said that he thought he used it to say "message received" or "I hear you." And, he admitted, sometimes he used it to stop the story-teller and redirect him or her. In that guise, "OK" meant "shut up." A word so ambiguous is dangerous and it is disconcerting to hear your doctor say "OK" when he means, "I hear you, please go on with your story" especially if you have just told him how bad you feel: "feeling weaker," or about a truly nasty diagnosis: "leukemia." Nor is it a good idea to use the little acronym to stop the patient or spouse in mid-speech any more than it would be therapeutic to tell them to "shut up".

What could this doctor do? He could say "I got you" or "I understand" or just nod to indicate reception. And when he wishes to interrupt and redirect the conversation, he could say, "I'm sorry, but I have to interrupt. I need you to go back to talking a little more about ..." Much more wordy, but also more polite.

Dr. Perch missed a number of opportunities for empathic responses during his conversation with this patient and his spouse. When we spoke of those opportunities, Dr. P. remarked that he had been aware of the significance of his patient's utterances, but didn't know what to say. That's pretty good; it is the first step in empathy. I divide the empathic response into three steps. One first notices that something remarkable was said. That's where Dr. Perch is. Then, the interviewer pauses and considers the statement. It helps me to ask myself, "How could this person be feeling to say what he just said to me?" Finally, the doctor has to tell the patient that he understands just how it felt. This communication provides a great deal of relief to the patient, simply letting our patient know that we understand how he feels.

Where might Dr. P. have used this sort of empathic tool? After being told the diagnosis, acute myelocytic leukemia, the doctor could have responded, "That must have been an ominous sort of thing to hear." Or "That would have been a scary piece of news, I imagine."

After being told about the doctors not being available when the patient was deteriorating and seeking help, the doctor might say, "Was it pretty frightening to be so ill and not able to find your doctors?" Of course, the patient might correct him, "Not so frightening as much as it made me angry." Then the doctor can amend to, "I understand. You felt angry when the doctors were all away just when you needed them."

And after the patient's wife described how she needed to extract stringy mucous from his mouth, the doctor might have wondered how this strong, independent rancher felt about being so weak and so dependent. "That must have felt awful to be so weak and so dependent." Or, he could consider the patient's wife. How did she feel? Perhaps he could try: "That must have been hard for you to see your husband so weak." Or, "I see that you are very devoted to one another."

Later on in the conversation not included in the fragment above, this same patient told his doctor that he knew two people at home who had recently died of leukemia. The doctor passed by this bit of news quickly. He missed an opportunity to ask his patient about thoughts of dying.

I think Dr. P. is close to the point of capitalizing on these conversational opportunities. He already can point to the affect-laden moments. Now he just needs to pause, reflect on the affective content, and give the patient some understanding that he, the doctor, really heard what was just said. When he does so, he will find his therapeutic relationships markedly strengthened, his patients happier, and his own pleasure magnified.

# I AN ALK I-OU I EEH

Phone call:   M: Dr. Platt? This is MacHeath, the resident at Presbyterian. I have a patient who just came in through the emergency room. She's in pretty bad heart failure. She needs a medical attending. Would you be able to take her on?

P: Sure, Mac.  Where is she now?

M: I have her on 2 center. I got a chest x-ray and the cardiogram and some labs.  Do you want to hear about her?

P: Sure, but I have a few minutes right now. How about if I walk across the street and come see her. Can I meet you at her bedside?

M: Great! I'll be there.

[Five minutes later, at the bedside]

P: Hello, Mrs. Robins. I'm Dr. Platt.

R: (an elderly woman with a gauze bandage covering her nose and midface) e-O. I ad oo EE u.

M: I didn't get time to tell you. She had a nasal carcinoma and had a resection.

P: I see. Mrs. Robins, can you tell us again what sort of trouble brought you to the emergency room today?

R: Eh. I oo-n eeh.

P: I'm having trouble understanding you.

M: That's right. I couldn't understand her. I mostly got my history from the old chart.

P: That probably won't help much with current symptoms.

R: I an alk i-ou I eeh.

P: What? Can you say that again?

R: EH. I AN ALK I-OU I EEH!

P: You can't talk without your teeth?

R: Eh.

P: I see. Where are your teeth?

R: I Y urs.

P: In your purse?

R: Eh.

P: Where is your purse?

R: O-eh ehh.

[She points to the bedside cabinet. Dr. M. opens the cabinet, retrieves the purse, and hands it to her. She reaches into her purse and removes a palate prosthesis with dentures. She places them into her mouth, jiggles them around a little, and then speaks.]

R: (nasal tone) That's better. What was it you wanted to know?

P: I wanted to know about the symptoms that got you to our emergency room today.

R: Oh, that's right. I was getting awfully short of breath. I couldn't breathe. It had been going on for days but was really bad last night.

## DISCUSSION

This resident, a very good physician already, somehow had managed to do the entire examination without asking about the communication difficulty. The patient's severe dysarthria was easily treated by returning her denture-palate prosthesis to its place. This interview occurred 15 years ago and Mac still remembers it to his chagrin.

It is funny that we sometimes ignore items that need attention and where a little bit of attention eases our work from then on. The approach to dealing with these disruptions is simply to share our problem with the patient. Sometimes there is no solution but one doesn't know until one tries to find out.

There is a second half to this interview. The resident, a bit unnerved by having been caught out over the conversational problem, was standing on one side of the bed while I, standing on my side began my physical examination. I removed the 4X4 that had been covering her midface. She had the result of major facial cancer surgery, a missing nose and an obvious opening through which one could see the posterior nasopharynx. The view was spectacular. Dr. MacHeath, looking into the gaping cavern, gasped "Oh my God!"

Later, out of the room,

P: Mac -

M: I know, I know. It just tumbled out of me.

As, indeed, it did. Perhaps not the best comment to make to a patient, since a lot of our reassurance consists of our own unflappability in the face of really nasty and really scary conditions, some of our own making.

Nonetheless, despite these technical problems, the patient did well. She improved under Dr. MacHeath's care of her heart failure. And Mac still remembers and still acts on his memory.

# PLEASE STEP THIS WAY

(Thanks to Dr. Philip R. Corsello)

As Dr. Corsello tells it, he had suffered a long tiresome day. Nothing went right. He was late to see his last patient, a person new to him, and he had no flexibility or forbearance left. The office suite consisted of a long string of examination rooms off a central hallway. One exam room, the one Dr. Corsello's new patient was seated in, had two doors, one to the suite hallway and one opening up to the outside office building hallway and serving as the suite's backdoor.

Dr. C: Hello. I'm really sorry to be so late. I know I've kept you waiting. I usually don't let this happen but today has been overwhelming. Anyway, now that I'm here, what can I do for you?

Mr. X: (A stern, angry-appearing man is silent.)

C: I can see that you're upset and I am sorry I'm late but, anyway, what sort of trouble have you been having?

X: You doctors are all the same! You think you are the only ones who are important. I have things to do too. Your time isn't the only time that matters. I don't even know if I want you to examine me.

C: You don't think you want me to examine you?

X: No.

C: Well. (stands) Then please step this way. (opens door to the outside hallway)

X: (goes through doorway)

C: I think you had better consult another doctor. Goodbye. (closes door)

## DISCUSSION

This story is a treasure to Dr. Corsello fifteen years after it took place. He is usually a peaceloving, nonconfrontive person and this sort of interaction was and is a rarity for him. He remembers the event as a true failure in doctor-patient communication but a small triumph over life and its pressures.

Nonetheless, one could consider other possible outcomes. For example, after the patient's "You doctors are all the same" speech, Dr. C. might have tried:

C: Umm. You've had other bad experiences with other doctors?
(planning to wait, to listen, and to invest some time needed to repay for the damage done)

The patient might respond:

X: You bet. The last doctor I saw just wanted to peddle his pills. He was always changing my prescriptions and never had time to listen to me.

C: You never felt you were getting the time you needed.

X: Right. And when I got worse, instead of working on it, he sends me to you.

C: And I keep you waiting forever in this little room.

X: Yeah. No one even told me how long you'd be.

C: Not a very good beginning. I can see how you'd be irritated.

X: Yeah. But I guess you guys have other problems than me. Sorry I bit your head off, Doc.

C: Well, we're even then. How about if we go back and start over? Can you tell me about your health problems?

It seems that Dr. C. was finished apologizing to his patient but his patient wasn't done with being angry. Simultaneity is hard to find in medical practice, as it is in other relationships. When we're ready for the medical story, our patient may not yet be. Then we must be patient to discover his story and his concerns.

R.C. Smith and R.B. Hoppe [7] distinguish between the patient's story, full of feelings, hopes, fears, and theories and the doctor's story, full of symptoms and organic-medical data. They make it clear that we need to hear the patient's story first and then make a gradual transition to the other data we want.

This patient needed first to tell us about his fears and experiences in encounters with doctors.

Dr. C. might have tried another tack. He was really tired and out of patience. He might have recognized that, shared it with the patient, and tried for another meeting.

C: I can sure see how distressing this must be for you and how aggravated you would be. I can see you not being sure whether you should trust me at all at this point. And the sad news is that I am really exhausted after a long hard day and I don't know if I have anything in myself to give to you. I wonder if we could make a new arrangement. For example, could I get you to come back tomorrow when I can be fresh and helpful and even on time? I would, of course, not charge you for today and to pay for my lateness today I would see you tomorrow too at no charge. Then we could have a fresh start and do a lot better together. What do you think?

When we really can't be doctors anymore, when we've spent all our resources, we have to admit it and ask for a rematch.

# *I CAN UNDERSTAND HOW YOU FEEL*

Dr. Cornea: Hello, Mrs. Groan, how are you doing?

Mrs. G: Not so good, Doctor. It's been two weeks since my operation and I am not getting better. My eye is still very red and it hurts. I didn't know it was going to keep hurting like this. My friend, Alice, had an operation on her eye and she was fine in three or four days. I just don't seem to be getting better. I'm kind of sorry I had the operation at all. I think I was better off before.

C: (leaning forward, speaking aggressively and forcibly) I can understand how you feel, but I think you just have to be more patient. These things take a little while to resolve and we often see post-operative inflammation that lasts several weeks. You just have to be willing to wait a little while longer and keep using the drops I prescribed. It helps to put them in every four hours just as I told you. I have examined your eyes several times and they are doing just fine. There is no reason for you to be concerned. All you have to do is use those drops just as I have told you. This little bit of inflammation is quite acceptable after an operation and I see nothing remarkable in my examination. It doesn't do any good to be impatient and your friend's clinical course has nothing to do with your condition. She might not even have had the same operation.

I don't see any reason for you to bring her into the discussion. And I don't think you have to be worried or upset. This is just part of the operative course and you have to let time do its work.

## DISCUSSION

Many of our most frustrating encounters with patients occur when the patient feels angry or sad and we are uncomfortable hearing about that bad feeling. Often it sounds as if we are being blamed for something. Often we *are* being blamed for something. It really is hard for the doctor. This is a tough challenge! Best is first to realize our own feelings. We can't easily deal with the patient's feelings until we own our own. We need to realize that we are feeling blamed, that we feel angry or resentful or sad. Sometimes we have to discuss this with the patient but usually we just need to sit with the feeling for a few moments, then consider how the patient might be feeling.

Then empathy is usually the best and most effective tool to use in such a situation. The first steps of an empathic statement require us to identify the patient's feeling, tell her clearly that we understand, supporting our claim by repeating her feelings, then *stop*. We are inclined to rush on to some sort of solution — to reassurance, explana-tion, direction, whatever. But what is called for is simply understand-ing. And, after understanding, a pause helps immeasurably. Wait for the patient to tell us what to do next. And even when the patient sug-gests our next move, we should not be in a hurry to get on with it — the opportunity to evince understanding is too valuable to let pass quickly.

So this doctor who was feeling unappreciated and blamed could have made a serious effort to let her patient know that she did under-stand how the patient felt. She could have stopped, perhaps said, "Let me think about what you've just said for a moment," allowing herself to think about how it must feel to the patient. Then she might have essayed a response such as, "Let me see. I can imagine that you are feeling worried right now. You are concerned that your eye is still red and painful. You are worried that perhaps something wasn't done right and you are even wondering if you should have had the eye operation or if you should have consulted a different eye doctor. That must feel really worrisome and frightening for you right now." She could add "you have a friend who seemed to get better much quicker and that worries you, too. You are not sure you are going to get better ever and are imagining all sorts of horrible complications. Is that the way it feels?"

Then, most important, she should not accept the temptation to rush into explanations, reassurances, or exhortations. Just stay with the understanding of how the patient is feeling. The patient will give hints of what to do next.

The patient might, for example, respond to the doctor with, "Yes, doctor, that is how I've been feeling. I know I have to be patient and just use the drops as you've told me, but it is hard not to be fright-ened." If so, all the doctor has to do is agree. "I can understand how you would be frightened. It is natural to feel that way. But I am glad to hear that you are using the eye drops. I agree that you need to be patient a little longer."

Or the patient might ask, "What is it you want me to do? I know you told me, but I've been so worried that I've forgotten your explana-tions." Again, our next task is clearly indicated by the patient. And all because we gave the patient to know that we understand how she feels.

My point is the immense therapeutic power of an empathic statement. It immediately eases the patient's sense of isolation. The doctor is *with* her patient. Anger, loss, and sadness all diminish when treated with empathy. We mustn't fail to use this most powerful tool. And we should learn to recognize the affect of the patient as a gift. The patient's fear or sadness or anger tells us immediately how she is feeling and gives us an easy entry. If we look at that affect as a gift to us rather than a threat, we can find the apt empathic statement to treat it with.

"I can understand how you feel" should be followed by our statement of what we have understood the patient's feelings to be. It is not a mechanical phrase, but rather the beginning of the most comforting therapeutic message we can give. Such a transaction needs thought and care and then its reward will be great for doctor and patient alike.

# DILAUDID

Phone operator: Doctor Smith, I have a patient of Dr. Wilson's on the phone. He says that he needs something right away for his terrible migraine. Can I patch him through for you?

Dr. S: I guess so. What is his name?

P.O.: He says he is Tom Hale.

S: OK, put him on.

Hello, this is Dr. Smith. Is this Mr. Hale?

H: Hall, Doctor, I'm Tim Hall. I used to be a patient of George Wilson's. He's an old friend of mine. Are you covering for him?

S: Yes, I am. What's up?

H: Oh, I'm sorry to bother you on Saturday night. I have these terrible migraines. George called them cluster headaches. They come on for a couple of weeks and then I'm OK again. I'm visiting family here in Denver and the headaches just started up again. I'm in terrible pain. George used to give me a couple of weeks of Dilaudid and that would be a big help. If I went over to the emergency room would you call them and ask them to have a prescription for me? I would have called George but I didn't have his home number with me.

S: I see. Well Dr. Wilson is out of town anyway this weekend.

H: That's OK. I'm sure you can take care of it. I usually get about 30 tablets of two milligrams. I could stop at St. Joes or Presbyterian, whichever you thought best.

S: Well, Mr. Hall, I'm not really very comfortable with that. I've never seen you before and I usually don't prescribe Dilaudid.

H: I can understand, doc. But George just gives me the prescription because he knows it works for me.

## DISCUSSION

Well, now, what have we here? Are you being conned into prescribing a narcotic that you don't want to prescribe? Why not? Would you prescribe it if you knew the patient? Not even then? Are you going to anger and alienate your colleague when he returns on Monday and learns how you treated his good friend?

Would you like to avoid getting up to go into the hospital? Do you suspect that this man only waited until late Saturday evening to catch you in a vulnerable state? Is it even possible for you to get him such a prescription without coming to meet him?

I guess that you are trapped. You have to make an offer and the easiest usually is to offer to meet him at the emergency room.

S: Mr. Hall, I can't do what you are asking. In fact, I almost never prescribe Dilaudid for migraine. If you want, I will come and meet you at the emergency room if you are in severe pain right now. Perhaps we can find something to give you some relief tonight. Unless I find a contrary problem when I examine you, I might be able to give you enough Dilaudid or some other pain medicine to last you through the weekend.

H: Oh for heaven's sake, Doctor. I'm not some sort of drug addict.

S: I understand. However, that is all I can do. Do you want to come to the emergency room and meet me there?

H: If you're not going to help me, I don't see any reason to make the trip. I'll just bear it until George comes back.

# *THEY MISTREATED ME AGAIN*

Dr. Smith:  Hello, Bill, how are you?

B:  Well, not so hot, Doctor. I laid one on. I really got drunk for a couple of days. But I've only had one drink today.

S:  My goodness. You were doing so well. How come?

B:  They mistreated me again. I got laid off. They called me in and said they were cutting down and I was laid off. I was just about to have a vacation and I had all sorts of plans.

S:  When was that?

B:  Just last week. So I said, "Fuck it" and I went out and got drunk.

S:  How did you feel?

B:  I was really angry. But after a couple of drinks I got calmed down. I figured, "What the hell?"

S:  So you were really angry.

B:  Yeah. I've been working for them for three years. I worked up from janitor to mechanic and stationary engineer and all that good work didn't go for nothing.

S:  Sounds like you were feeling unappreciated and hurt, too.

B:  Yeah. I know I shouldn't drink. You showed me all those tests on my liver and how it was messed up. But they mistreated me and I just said "To hell with it."

S:  So they mistreat you and then you go and mistreat yourself, too. That's sort of double punishment.

B:  Yeah, I guess so.

S:  I can understand that, but now I think you ought to stop again and get back on the wagon.

B:  Yeah, I know I should.

S:  Because you are really doing yourself harm if you keep drinking.

B:  Yeah, Doc. The thing is, they messed me up. I was doing OK and they treated me like shit.

S:  That must have been terrible. But now it's time to stop again.

B:  Yeah.

# DISCUSSION

This doctor does listen to his patient and does give empathic support. Probably he is being helpful. However, at the end he wants to tell the patient what to do and hopes that his patient will just follow his recommendations.

Statistics on adherence to our recommendations are dismal.[L] Only about 50% of patients follow the doctor's recommendations and the percentage is far less when a behavioral disorder such as alcoholism is the problem. And this patient gives strong hints that he will not follow recommendations because he views himself as a victim and is not in the business of taking responsibility for himself. He has no inkling why he was fired even though perhaps his drinking had something to do with it. He sees himself as a mistreated victim.

Some of my alcoholic patients describe their drinking as if it were a metter of chance rather than a matter of choice.

Dr. F: Are you going to stop drinking? Are you going to continue?

Pt. X: I don't know, Doc, it depends on what happens.

F: What do you mean?

X: Well, if I bump into some buddies and they ask me to have a drink, I'll probably have a drink. If not, I probably won't.

I call that the rain theory of alcoholism. If you go outside and it is raining, you will probably be rained on. You don't have a lot of control over the weather. Some drinkers view their drinking as just as uncontrolled. But to get a handle on it, to achieve any control over any behavior, the patient has to assume responsibility and make active decisions. Bill doesn't sound as if he has reached that realization. If not, no amount of exhortation by the doctor is likely to do any good. What the doctor needs to do is stay with the responsibility issue.[23]

Dr. S: Bill, I can understand how you were feeling bad, angry and despondent, and came apart and started to drink again. Now you have to decide what you are going to do next. Nobody else can make that decision for you. You know that the drinking eases your feelings of anger and sadness, and you know that you are killing yourself by drinking. I guess you have your future in your own hands.

B: I suppose, Doc. But they sure have been messing with my mind.

S: Yes, they have. And you have, too. What you do now is up to you, though.

B: Yeah, I guess I have to decide what I'm going to do.

S: I agree.

B: I could just go back and keep drinking.

S: True.

B: Maybe I ought to stop. Can you give me some Librium again for the next few days?

S: Yes, I can. I'd be glad to try to help you if you choose to stop drinking. I'm not much help if you keep drinking, though. Let's talk a little more about stopping. As I understand it, you have conflicting desires. You see alcohol as your problem and also as your support system. What do you know about quitting? Have you done it before?

B: I did quit, three times before.

S: Any troubles with quitting?

B: Not really, some nausea and the shakes.

S: So if you decide to stop, you can.

B: Yeah, I guess I will.

S: OK, Bill, I am glad to hear that. I do believe you can do it. You did it before and I think you can again. Let's try a bit of the Librium to tide you over and perhaps you can come back in a few days and tell me how you're doing. I have confidence in you, but if you have trouble, I'd like to know. Can you come back Friday?

B: OK, Doc, I'll do that.

# JUST DIZZY

Vern:  Doc, I'm having a terrible time with this dizziness. You got to give me something for it.

Dr. Kindly:  Well, Vern, tell me more about it. How are you dizzy?

V: Just dizzy, Doc. I get dizzy and I just don't feel good.

K:  What do you mean, dizzy?

V:  Dizzy. I mean just dizzy. My head is just not right.

K:  Some people mean different things by "dizzy." Do you mean you feel faint? That the room is turning? That you feel lost in space? What?

V:  Yeah, that's it. All of them.

K:  Oh me. Have you fainted?

V:  No, not quite. I might though.

K:  Fallen? Do you fall?

V:  No, but I have to hold on to things.

K:  So you feel as if you might faint. Does your vision grey out or do you get sweaty?

V:  No, none of them, Doc, just dizzy.

K:  How have you been otherwise?

V:  Fine, Doc. Except for the dizziness I feel fine.

K:  Down in the dumps? Depressed?

V:  No, just dizzy. Look, Doc, I'm just dizzy. Can't you just give me something for it?

## DISCUSSION

Common things are common, even if we wish they weren't. Dizziness is one of the two most common presenting symptoms in a neurologist's practice, along with headache, and one of the ten most common in an internist's. We need to have some sense of how to approach this common problem, often aggravated by the patient's belief that he has a simple problem and it ought to have a simple solution.

Dr. Martin Samuels says that dizzy patients fit into four categories: a) faint and fainting, b) vertiginous, c) lacking proprioception and thus at sea in space, d) "just dizzy." He thinks that the last category is usually equivalent to depression and should be treated as such. I'm not sure about the depression equivalent but sure do recognize the "just dizzy" category.

This patient's physical examination can be expected to be quite normal. And we can predict that he will not benefit from most treatments. It might not be a bad idea to try an antidepressant. At the very least, such therapy will probably provoke a postural hypotension that will produce a new sort of dizziness that we can treat by stopping the drug.

What to do with the patient's insistence that he has a simple problem and can be easily treated? I see nothing but a straightforward explanation.

Dr. K:  Vern, I know that you think this dizziness is a pretty simple problem and ought to be easily treated. Unfortunately I have to tell you that we aren't anywhere that clever about dizziness. We find it a very confusing symptom and one that is very hard to treat. Often nothing we do is much help. The symptom can be very bothersome and yet never do you any more harm and often we can't do much to help it. That must sound very annoying to you.

V:  Yeah, Doc, it does. You mean you can't do something about it?

K:  Not much.

V:  That doesn't sound right. There ought to be something you could do.

Unfortunately honest explanations don't always satisfy. But the patient's lack of satisfaction gives us a chance to try to be empathic.

K:  I can understand how you feel. You think you have a simple problem and that we ought to have a simple solution for you. It must be very frustrating for you to find that we don't.

V:  Damn right! I come here for some help and you arent going to do anything. Maybe I ought consult a specialist.

Unfortunately empathy may not be enough either. Thank goodness, there are specialists whose very function is not knowing what to do about dizziness.

K: I think that might be a very good idea. There are two sorts of specialists who deal with these problems even more often than I do, ear doctors and nerve doctors. I haven't found them to be much help for my patients who suffer from this sort of dizziness but you might feel a lot better just for having consulted such a doctor. What would you like to do?

V: Well, to tell you the truth, Doc, what I'd like is for you to just give me something to help with the dizziness.

K: Vern, there are a lot of medicines that have been tried in this sort of problem. We can use one that is often helpful, and then see how you are doing in a week. Sometimes the medicine is helpful only after a longer period, perhaps two weeks. OK?

V: OK.

# WHY DID YOU COME
# TO THE HOSPITAL?

Dr. Quell: Hello, Mrs. Mann, I'm Dr. Quell.

M: Hello Doctor.

Q: I need to go over you and help your doctor sort things out. First, would you tell me why you came to the hospital?

M: The doctor wanted me to come. I didn't. So I went home. My husband is next door to dialysis so I wanted to be home. Then today he made me come back.

Mr. Mann: She didn't improve any.

Q: Why did you go to the doctor?

M: Because Dr. Graham was on vacation. So I went to see his partner, Dr. Gilroy.

Q: Huh. Maybe I better ask it differently. Tell me how you came here.

M: Oh, my husband drove us. He isn't as good a driver as he used to be.No, really, Dear, you aren't, you know. It's his eyes. They aren't right since the diabetes. But we got here even if we're a little slower. We parked in the big garage and came through the bridge into the hospital. That used to be the admissions place but now, with all that building they're doing, we had to go down to the basement to register. It's really quite confusing.

Q: You aren't kidding. What I mean is I need to know what's the matter with you.

Mr. M: Hell, I've been married to her for 35 years. I could tell you plenty on that score.

M: He's just joking. He's been worried about me. Of course, we both worry about each other. What was it you wanted to know?

Q: What's the trouble that brought you here?

M: Well, I had polio when I was a young woman. I've never been right since.

# DISCUSSION

This is circumstantiality at its best. Sometimes doctors call such patients tangential but I like to differentiate tangential story tellers from circumstantial ones. A tangential talker goes farther and farther from the subject, eventually getting so far away that neither he nor the interlocutor know how he got there. This circumstantial talker stays roughly the same distance from the center of her tale, never getting closer or farther. And she tells the circumstances of everything, not the thing itself.

A second danger presents if we get her to talk about the illness, for she is likely to switch gears to medical circumstances. Then she will talk about the doctors, the diagnoses, the tests, and the therapies. She will tell a saga of medical care that will sound like a medical history but really be just a pseudo-history.

Q: I need you to tell me more about this illness you are having now.

M: Oh, well Dr. Graham says it is sarcoidosis. He says the chest x-ray shows an interstitial shadow and that there are big lymph nodes. He checks my oxygen in my finger every time I come in. Last week it was lower than ever and he said that maybe I need another lung biopsy. The last time, about five years ago, Dr. Lunger put his long bronchoscope down into my lungs and took a piece out. The trouble is I got a collapsed lung and they had to put a big tube in my side. They've treated me with antibiotics and Ceftin and prednisone and they don't know what to do. They said maybe they'd ask a big lung expert here at the hospital, Dr. Breath, to see me. So I guess I'm here so everyone can have a stab at me.

Again, although this sounds more medical than her parking garage story, it is lacking in any primary data, lacking symptoms. We have no idea *how* she is not well and no time course for the symptoms that we have yet to meet. If she has an illness other than sarcoidosis, we are not going to make a diagnosis this way. We need to ask her to focus on symptoms.

Q: Mrs. Mann, I really need your help here. For a few minutes I need you to tell me just about you, nothing about what your doctors did or said. I need understand the exact symptoms you've been having.

M: Symptoms? OK, let's see. I guess the main thing is that I just don't have any energy. I get tired after any least little thing. I'm OK in the morning when I get up but then I get so very tired by noon and I'm no good at all in the afternoon.

Q: Uh huh?

M: And Dr. Graham says that the oxygen is low, but that isn't enough to explain and...

Q: No, Mrs. Mann, please go on with your symptoms. Besides the fatigue, anything else?

M: Well, I've been having diarrhea. Sometimes my bowels are awfully dark. And I get short of breath, of course, but that's just about the way it's been for years. Dr. Graham says... Oh, that's right, you just want to know how I feel. Well, aside from tired and short-winded and the diarrhea, OK, I guess.

Q: Huh! Tell me more about this diarrhea. And what did you mean "awfully dark?"


I should note that nothing brings out the circumstantiality as much as a question about circumstances. So this doctor might cultivate some other opening queries rather that his "Why did you come to the hospital" or, even worse, "How did you come to the hospital?", a question that is all too often answered, "in my car."

Dr. Gordon wonders if this patient has an organic brain syndrome. Could be! However I believe that many people fail to satisfy the definitions of organic brain disorders but still have bizarre and non-productive communication styles. We all know friends and relatives who cannot answer a simple question any way but with a pageant. Tangential and circumstantial speakers abound and may be undisciplined but need not be confused.

# I CAN'T MAKE YOU UNDERSTAND

Dr. Hill:  So you have been feeling tired, Mrs. Smith?

S: Yes, Doctor. I just don't seem to ever get any better.

H: And this has been going on since your divorce?

S: I wake up tired and I go to bed tired. There's nothing but tired all day. And I ache all over. I have pain everywhere.  Everything hurts all the time.

H: What hurts the most?

S: Everything hurts, Doctor, everything. And I'm so weak and I get dizzy all the time.

H: Is there anything that hurts more than anything else?

S: I told you, Doctor, everything hurts. I just can't seem to be able to make you understand.

H: Well perhaps you could just answer my question.

S: What question? Everything hurts and I'm always tired. I'm sorry, I'm not explaining this very well.

H: No, you're not. You should try to focus on one thing at a time. What, for example, is the worst symptom?

S: I don't know. I probably shouldn't waste your time.

H: You're not wasting my time.

S: Yes, well, maybe I don't have anything wrong. You said that the tests were all normal.

H: That's true.

S: But I feel so bad all the time.


## DISCUSSION

I think this case demonstrates the vagueness of symptomatology in depression, almost surely the diagnosis. The patient is really being very specific in her inspecificity. But it also shows the distress the patient feels about her job of explaining to the doctor. She is really struggling to do this. Will she, a relatively uneducated person, ever be able to explain how she feels to this exalted hyper-educated person who hardly speaks her language? Many patients have such fears and uncertainties. Most patients are already anxious about their ability to do what is needed in the doctor's office. It is common to have your patient say, somewhere in the interview, "I just can't explain it to you." That usually presents a golden opportunity for you to respond that he or she is doing just fine.

"You're doing a good job explaining it. Please continue."

Even if the patient is presenting less than a fully coherent story, such support usually helps. It decreases anxiety and allows the process to go on.

Nonetheless, this patient is frustrating to her doctor. He finds it hard to cope with her imprecision, maybe even wants to punish her for it. He could stop to consider his own feelings, probably an essential step before trying to consider hers. How can we understand her if we don't yet understand ourselves? If we do realize our own feelings and still are puzzled by the patient, we can say so.

"I'm sorry, but I'm hopelessly confused. Can you help me understand better?" A request for help from the patient after owning our own confusion does wonders. Of course we must avoid suggestions that the patient is at fault. Any blaming usually meets with denial or counterattack. It is not helpful to suggest that the patient is inadequate at explaining his or her problem to you and to do so might lead to worsening of the relationship. If you are having trouble understanding, the best device to use is gentle, nonjudgmental confrontation that allows you to own the problem and the patient to assist you with clarification.

# SOMEONE ELSE KNOWS

Dr. Smith:  Tell me more about the nausea.

Ms. Teak:  My pharmacist said I might try lying down.

S:  Lying down? Did that help?

T:  I don't know, I didn't try it.

S:  Well, did you notice any relationship between position or activity and your symptoms?

T:  I didn't, but my husband thought I probably shouldn't do any more work in the garden. He thought it might bring on the nausea.

S:  Is that true? Did it?

T:  Oh I really can't tell. I haven't done any gardening for weeks.

S:  So what did seem to make your trouble worse?

T:  I didn't notice anything, Doctor. I really don't know. But my daughter thought it was probably something I ate.

S:  Sounds as if everyone has a hypothesis except for you.

T:  I guess so. But you know, sometimes I don't know and someone else does. That's why I come to a doctor.

S:  Touché.


What's going on?

How do you get the patient to tell you what *you* most need to know to make a diagnosis? Is there a conflict here with what the *patient* needs to tell you?


## DISCUSSION

How touching the confidence that people place in others. Thank goodness for it. It explains our patients' trust in us. Sometimes it is quite surprising though. And it is always a trial to our patience to see if we can stand hearing the stories and hypotheses of third parties.

One of my favorite examples occurs when a patient comes to me from another doctor, having lost confidence in that doctor and desiring a new opinion:

Mr. Jones: I've been going to Dr. Brown for years but he just isn't getting anywhere with this problem. I think he's getting old and maybe not keeping up anymore. I don't think he is such a good diagnostician anymore.

P: I see. What sort of trouble have you been having?

J: Well, Dr. Brown says it is chronic bronchitis.

P: And how is it bothering you?

J: Dr. Brown says it is aggravating my gall bladder.

Even having lost confidence in Dr. Brown's diagnostic acumen, the patient cannot avoid telling you everything Dr. Brown thought or said.

The challenge for me is to stay calm and not lose my patience. I often try to get the patient to talk about symptoms, but I'm not always successful. Dr. Smith might try this with Ms. Teak.

S: Ms. Teak, it would really help me if we could leave those helpful people out for a moment and just understand what you noticed about your symptoms. You said that you were troubled with nausea, no pain, no vomiting. I need to understand just when and where the nausea appeared.

T: OK, Doctor. I remember that my husband thought I was complaining mostly when the television was on. He wondered if I was getting some sort of radiation.

S: And what did you notice?

T: I'm getting to that, doctor. He thought those reruns were the worst.

See? Sometimes it doesn't work. Besides, maybe we really need to hear something else from the patient. Mishler [K] might say that we are hearing the voice of the life-world. People tell stories, not symptoms, and they assign meaning and cause to everything. They tie events together. And they ask others for help. By the time a patient comes to us, she may have discussed her problems with several others.

This doctor might try returning to this other aspect of the patient's story. Perhaps it could go like this:

S: I can see that you've discussed your illness with several other people.

T: Sure. Wouldn't anybody?

S: Hmm. (nod a bit)

T: It's pretty scary to just go to a doctor.

S: Sure.

T: I remember my aunt. She had a bad stomach, too; eventually it led to cancer.

S: (nod)

T: I thought I could, it could...

S: Maybe be sick like her?

T: Yeah.

S: So it was pretty scary to come here.

T: Yeah.

S: How about now?

T: Well I feel OK, I guess.

S: Let's come back to this later. For now, could you help me understand the symptoms you've been having? Pain? Nausea? Shortness of breath? Cough? Whatever?

T: Well, mostly the nausea, I guess. It woke me most every morning about seven and a couple of times I had to vomit. Later, after I ate a cracker or two, it got better.


Now we're doing better. Somehow we need to find room for both voices, that of the life world and that of medicine.

# WHAT ARE THE SYMPTOMS
# OF LIVER CANCER?

Lisa: Dr. Platt, what are the symptoms of diabetes?

P: Well, usually a great thirst, lots of urinating, and weight loss despite a very good appetite and intake.

L: I would imagine that you would urinate a lot if you drank a lot because of a great thirst.

P: That's true. But in diabetes the sequence goes the other way; you lose a lot of urine, get dehydrated, and then have to drink to keep up. Why do you ask?

L: Because Steve says I get really mean if I haven't eaten for a while. And I do. I have to eat when I am hungry or I get all tired and cranky. We were walking in the mountains and I said, "Steve, let's stop. I want to eat something." And he said that it would be better to go on for ten minutes more until we got to a nice spot to picnic. But I was hungry just then. I got very angry when he wouldn't stop.

P: So why not carry something to munch on yourself? Why make yourself dependent on Steve? I'd get angry too. I can imagine doing that to my wife. She would refuse to go a foot farther if I didn't stop for food when she wanted it. Why not carry your own food?

L: I should, but sometimes in the packing of backpacks, all the food goes in one.

P: OK, Lisa, so far I hear that when you get hungry you are cross and want to eat just then. Anything else?

L: No, but I wondered if that could be diabetes.

P: I don't think so. We could check your blood sugar but we'd have to catch you feeling that way. All your blood tests have been normal up to now.

L: Well, OK. Then I should tell you that about five weeks ago I had pain for a day or two in my left side, right over the shoulder blade. Then it hurt up in the front of my chest, above my left breast. I talked with a friend of mine, an old German doctor, and he asked if I ate much fat. I said that I didn't and he suggested that I eat some ham and eggs. So I ate some eggs and the pain went away. He thinks maybe I have stones in my gallbladder.

P: Oh my goodness, this is more than I can take today. Lisa, sometimes I can hear this sort of thing and sometimes not. I think today isn't one of my best days. I'm afraid that the gallbladder is on the other side. Maybe I ought to hear more about your chest.

L: It isn't my chest I'm worried about. Besides, I know about referral pain. Sometimes it doesn't hurt where the problem is. I know that.

P: True. But the pain doesn't go clear across to the other side. No, left chest pain is usually caused by something in the chest and surely something on the left side.

L: Well, maybe so. Anyway the pain went away and I haven't had it for over a month. Besides, I'm worried about my gall bladder, my liver, and my pancreas. What are the symptoms of liver cancer?

P: You know, usually I try to work from the other direction—find out what symptoms you have and match the disease with them. So far I haven't heard anything from you that sounds like disease of those organs.

L: That may be, but I'm still worried. What do we have to do to be sure I don't have a cancer of the liver or the pancreas?

P: Why are you worried about that?

L: My mother and my mother's sister died of liver cancer.

P: Primary liver cancer? Or did it begin elsewhere like the breast or bowel or ovary?

L: No, it began in the liver. But they were all full of cancer when the diagnosis was made.

P: That's hard. I can imagine how frightening it must be for you. But unfortunately we don't have any simple test to screen for those cancers in early, treatable stages. Even if we did a CAT scan...

L: Yes, what about a CAT scan? We could do one every time I came in.

P: No we couldn't. That would be way too much radiation for one thing. And I haven't heard anything yet that would lead me to suggest even one CAT scan. Are you feeling sick? Are you having any symptoms now?

L: No, I feel pretty good. We went for a long hike last week and I did fine, even up at 12,000 feet. And I'm not depressed any more like I was last winter. No, I'm just worried about getting liver cancer or pancreas cancer and I would like you to test me for those two. I don't care if you haven't heard anything that would make you do a CAT scan. I want one done.

P: Oh me. This is ridiculous. We can't work that way. And it would be crazy to do periodic CAT scans. I don't even think they could detect liver cancer or pancreas cancer early enough to make a difference.

L: Well, what can we do to be sure I don't have one of those two?

# DISCUSSION

The obvious problem is that the patient has an agenda that doesn't match the doctor's. But then what? I think I was perilously close to really offending and driving away my patient. She was seriously concerned and I thought it was all a big joke. I thought it was a game called 'I'll think of the diagnosis and you tell me the symptoms'. I thought my patient was invading my side of the street, wanting to be the doctor. I wanted her to be the patient.

When asked how I had been feeling just prior to this interview, I remembered that it was a day I hoped to go on autopilot. I wasn't feeling adventurous and hoped everything would be easy and straightforward. I expected this patient to be exactly that way; she was familiar to me, quite healthy, had improved dramatically from a past depressive illness on my therapy, and should present no problem I couldn't address. Instead she came with serious concerns that I couldn't defuse and with a plan that seemed inappropriate to me.

I think that you do what you can on a given day and some days it is not much. If you have little inventiveness, little flexibility, little tolerance for human foibles on some days, it isn't surprising. But on those sorts of days you need to have fallback positions and processes; you need cushions to protect your patients and yourself from damage. The cushions include a long-standing relationship with the patient. A long term patient will tolerate your having a bad day better than a brand new one will.

You must apologize when called for. I spend a lot of time saying that I am sorry. This time I had to apologize. "I'm sorry that I am having a hard time hearing your serious concerns today. The story of the old German doctor who thought gall bladders might cause left chest pain touched my funny bone. I'm not at my best today."

Sometimes it helps to try to avoid saying too much. If you are likely to hurt your patient's feelings whatever you say, it's best to say nothing. And above all, slow down. If the flow seems to be getting away from you, slow down, think, try to imagine how this patient might be feeling to have just said what she said.

And finally, negotiate. Sometimes it doesn't even hurt to do something that isn't altogether sensible medically but satisfies the patient. You might be wrong some day, and you can be sure that when you are wrong, you will have just made some absolute statement such as "A CAT scan won't show a thing." If you are absolutely sure that the CAT scan will be useless but can't convince your patient of that logically, you had better be careful. My superstition tells me that will be the very time that the CAT scan will reveal a clear cut, well-demarcated, early, resectable cancer.

If you do not do it now, someone else will and you will first learn about it from an attorney representing your ex-patient.

So I did apologize, did negotiate, and did order the CAT scan. I said that I realized that I was not being very sensitive to her concerns and that I was sorry; that just wasn't my day to be sensitive. She allowed that everyone had such days. I said that I saw no reason to suspect visceral cancer but that I would do a biochemical survey and check a CEA level and once, just once, we could do a CAT scan if she would agree not to insist on repeat X-ray studies of that sort. She promised to be satisfied with one study. I didn't do much of a job about exploring her fears and why they were peaking just then. But we parted as allies and the possibility still exists for future exploration.

As expected, the CAT scan, biochemical survey, and CEA were all normal.

Maybe, on her next visit, we will be able to talk about her fears and what is going on in her life.

One more problem: I explain too much. That's probably why I'm writing this book. As a physician, I tend to be explaining when I should be listening or asking for clarification. I think I got too talkative with this patient and would have done much better if I could have restrained myself and let her tell me more. Next time I will try to be quiet. If she asks direct questions, I will try to answer more with requests for clarification and try to give fewer medical lectures.

# SIGN OUT AMA

The patient was 47 years old, hospitalized for a bout of acute pancreatitis. She was known to be a heavy drinker but had been dry for two years. The pancreatitis had begun three years ago, had been relatively quiescent for the last six months, then flared up. She smoked two packs of cigarettes daily, took a few acetaminophen tablets, and had no allergies. She lived alone, worked as a telephone operator, and had no other serious past illnesses. On two prior hospital admissions she had been difficult for the nursing staff, who found her to be demanding and uncooperative.

The phone call came 8PM Sunday night.

Dr. Xylom: Hello, this is Doctor Xylom.

R: Hello Doctor. This is Rene, the nurse on 2 west at St. Righthere. I'm calling to tell you that your patient, Mrs. Howitz, left AMA.

X: Left AMA? What? How did that happen? She was fine when I saw her this morning.

R: Well, nothing we could do seemed to satisfy her. And she kept smoking even though she was in a non-smoking room. We even took her cigarettes away. She just got more and more angry and finally nothing we could say convinced her to stay. We made her sign the AMA form though, so everything is OK.

X: Oh great! Then what? What is she going to do now? What arrangements did you make?

R: There wasn't any way we could arrange anything with her. When she said she was going home we told her you hadn't discharged her. She said that she didn't give a damn whether you or anyone else discharged her. We told her she couldn't continue to do things against hospital policy but that if she was leaving, she had to sign the AMA form. She said she'd be glad to sign it. So, anyway, she left.

X: I see. Un huh. OK. Is there anything you want from me now?

R: No, we just had to inform you.

X: OK, thanks.

# DISCUSSION

Whoever invented the 'Against Medical Advice' form could not have been a physician. What a crazy way to do business! Our job is to care for the patient and to do that we must negotiate, always use negotiation with our patients. What is the use of a form that forces the patients' backs up against the wall and obliges them to carry out their threats to leave? Besides, my medical attorney friends say that it is a worthless piece of paper, that what is needed is a clear note in the chart detailing the conversation we have with our patient. And if the patient is not competent to make sensible decisions, we can't just let her walk out of the hospital. We may need to use what is euphemistically called therapeutic restraint. We might have to tie her down to treat her until we can get her status clarified, a court order if necessary, an adjudication about competency made, perhaps a 72-hour hold. But this patient was quite competent. She and the nursing staff became tangled up in an escalating conflict of rules and desires, a true power struggle, until, to show that she was really the person in charge of her own body, she left the hospital. I suppose that the nurses showed her who was in charge of the ward and she showed them who was in charge of her body.

What is a better course? Someone, somewhere in the downhill spiral, could have engaged the patient in a negotiation. What is she willing to do? If leaving the hospital is the only step she can tolerate, will she agree to come to see her doctor in the office tomorrow? Will she come next week? If she doesn't have to leave the hospital, what arrangement can we negotiate that will be tolerable to her and to her nurses? If she can't smoke in her room, can we change rooms or roommates? If not, can we find a place in the hospital where she can smoke? If not, can we supply her with nicotine gum or patches?

I think that the AMA form only serves to hasten the patient's exodus. It is about as effective as a kick in the rear to move the patient out of our hospital. And it results in an angrier and less cooperative patient. She will never want to return to this hospital or perhaps to this doctor. If that is the nurses' goal, maybe it is a miraculous solution. But most often the doctor and the patient still have plenty of work to do and ought to do it. A patient's abrupt exit from the hospital avoids the problem.

Is there a characteristic patient personality type or psychiatric diagnosis that leads to power struggles like this? Although not universal, surely a number of patients who leave the hospital against medical advice fit the definition of the borderline personality disorder. Plagued with inappropriate and excessive anger and difficulty in relationships with other people, they often have trouble with hospital rules and staff attempts to set limits on behavior.

James Groves, writing of "borderline patients", says that these people "ruthlessly destroy the very care they crave and cannot tolerate paradox."[24]

Unfortunately this style often mobilizes further the nursing staff's desire to set limits and then there is escalation. As much as possible, we need to learn and use conflict resolution tools, not AMA forms.[25,26]

# STAFF ABUSE

Last month, after John Lewis had been seen in the office and had left for home, a delegation of office staff appeared in the doctor's office. They wanted him to know that John was abusive to them, that he made it very hard for them to work with him, and that they suspected he wasn't that way with the doctor.

Dr. Xylom: No, I never would have imagined it. What is it he does?

Fern: Well, last visit he stood at the desk and shouted at me. He called me insolent and said that I had insulted him by asking for payment.

Alice: And a couple of months ago he bumped my car when he parked. I asked him for his insurance since he had badly dented the bumper and he insisted that he hadn't done anything. When my insurance adjuster said it would cost over a hundred dollars, John said the damage must have been there before.

Diana: He came in and was very rude when we were going over his insurance papers. I told him that we would help him with them and he said that we could do it or not, it wasn't his worry, and it was just our money anyway.

Pat: He was kind of lewd with me. He hinted that we ought to get together somewhere else. He's old enough to be my grandfather almost.

X: Wow! I had no idea of any of this. How come nobody told me anything?

D: We just hadn't all talked together. Anyway, we thought you ought to know.

X: Yes, surely. I will have to talk to him about this. He can't be abusive to you; we can't tolerate it. He is always so nice with me, so appreciative and cooperative.

D: Yes, we thought so. But he's terrible with us.

X: I've cared for him for ten years. Is he always troublesome?

D: No, I think this is all a matter of the last few months. He wasn't so difficult before. He never did seem terribly friendly but he wasn't a trouble.

One month has now passed and John is coming in for his routine visit. He has chronic kidney disease and bad knees. He uses a walker, lives alone, but seems to have rather stable medical problems.

What are you going to say?


# DISCUSSION

First of all, you are lucky that your staff came to you and let you in on the problem. They might have elected to take matters into their own hands and wreak retribution on this patient. Second, you must support your staff. No one should be the victim of abusive behavior, not you and not your staff.

Several questions come up. Why is John behaving this way now? What has triggered this bad behavior? Is it some sort of organic brain pathology? Is it an emotional disturbance? An emotional illness? Is he feeling vulnerable and unlovable? Is it just a matter of cultural bad manners? Why doesn't he abuse you? Are you safe from it because of your power? Does he need you too much to chance affronting you? Is he really angry with you but, afraid of hitting out at you, does he dump his anger on your more defenseless staff? And how are you going to broach the subject with him?

One solution not available to you is to neglect the problem and hope it will go away. Your staff cannot tolerate such non-support. I suggest steeling yourself and putting the difficulty to your patient. This is how the conversation went:

Dr. Xylom: John, I have something I need to discuss with you. I am not quite sure how to approach the topic and will need some help from you. Several members of my staff have come to me to say that you seemed quite displeased with them and that you then treated them badly. I hadn't heard of it before and need you to fill me in.

John: Oh, I'm not really having any trouble with them, Bill. Just maybe with Fern. She is young enough to be my grand-daughter and she calls me John when she puts me in the room. I was going to say something but I didn't. Then one day I barely nudged her car and she came running out, claiming that I had dented it. I think she put one over on me.

X: Hmm. What else?

J: Nothing else. The others are all fine.

X: Well, John, several of my staff have felt mistreated, that you were angry with them and let them know it.

J: I might have. Sometimes I have a little trouble with my temper.

X: You know, if you are angry, you can come tell me. I'm able to hear that. But you mustn't punish my employees. If there is a problem, I have to do the work.

J: I know, Bill. I guess I've just been pretty irritable recently.

X: What's going on? What else is eating on you?

J: Nothing much. Of course, I don't have a very good relationship with my daughter and her family. They hardly ever call me or see me unless I call them. And my other daughter is too busy and farther away. And, since Irene died, I've been pretty much alone. Sometimes I get to thinking that nothing is worth much anymore.

X: I see. So you've really been pretty lonely and sometimes down in the dumps. And you think you're more irritable than usual for you.

J: That's right. I'm doing a little better now, but I was kind of blue for a few months. I didn't tell you because I thought that wasn't really your problem. You're my internist.

X: Are you still depressed?

J: No, I was never really depressed, more just grumpy. You know my way isn't to sit around feeling sorry for myself. I've started playing bridge again and I made some visits with my kids, all on my own, and it seems better now.

X: OK. Can we talk again for a moment about the staff here?

J: Sure.

X: I need your promise that you will tell me if anyone offends you, but that you won't take over my job of supervision.

J: That sounds fine. I'll tell you if there are any problems.


Subsequently, Dr. X. shared some of John's story of loneliness and sadness with the office staff. They agreed to use his last name, treating him as respectfully as possible. They agreed to report any difficult interactions immediately. Indeed, subsequent visits have gone swimmingly with no evident transgressions on either side.

# SHORTHAND

Melinda Sharp is a 50-year-old woman who has been hospitalized many times for a multitude of psychiatric diagnoses including bipolar affective disorder, schizophrenia, and borderline personality disorder. She comes to her internist monthly, always with a list of her problems written in shorthand. She immediately moves the examining room furniture in order to be able to face the doctor directly. As soon as the doctor enters the room she begins with her usual problem:

S: Doctor, my husband has been so terrible to me again. He beats me up and rips my clothes and calls me terrible names. He never used to be this way until he got his stomach cancer. Now he's just evil. I don't know what to do. I can't call the police as you suggested because they would arrest him and he'd have a record and he wouldn't forgive me. And he won't go to a psychiatrist or anyone.

This topic had been the subject of her last ten visits. At no time was there any evidence of traumatic damage, no scrapes or bruises. She always found reasons to explain why any suggestion I made wouldn't work.

I was at my wit's end. I thought I couldn't stand any more of these interactions. I told my wife of my difficulty that evening.

F: I don't know what to do with this patient. She pins me in the room, holds me with this interminable list that is in shorthand so I can't take it away and read it. She rearranges my furniture and has a litany of unchanging complaints that I can't do anything with.

Connie: Why do you continue to see her?

F: I feel obliged to. No one else cares for her and I feel that it is part of my work.

C: And by your description, you must feel quite oppressed by her.

F: That's it exactly. She is between me and the door. She has that list that I can't read and I want to get away the moment I get in the room.

C: Even her tales of being the victim of marital violence seem another oppression to you.

F: Not so much the tale as the unsolvability. She plays "Why Don't You? Yes, But..." with me.

C: Have you suggested that she tell the police about her husband's violence?

F: Several times.

C: Well, you might suggest that she talk with a Safehouse counselor.

F: That might help. Maybe she'll go play "Why Don't You?" with the counselor.

C: Or perhaps you might tell her that you just won't listen to her do nothing about a dangerous situation, that she has to take an action or stop telling about being victimized.

On the next visit, a carbon copy of the last, the patient began with her usual litany of complaints about her husband.

F: Melinda, I have to ask you to stop. I can't hear this any more.

M: But, Doctor, he is so brutal to me.

F: Melinda, stop. I have decided that I can't cope with this story any more. Either you report him to the police or stop telling me about him. In fact, I am going to refuse to hear any more complaints about how your husband treats you unless you call the local police in. If you don't, I can't be your doctor anymore.

M: I don't see how I can call in the police. And he is so evil, so hateful to me..

F: No, I mean it. You must stop.

M: But ...

F: No more.

M: You won't listen to me about him?

F: No.

M: I do want to keep you as my doctor. I guess I'll have to tell him that I am going to call the police. Can I use your phone?

The patient then called her husband and carried on an animated conversation with him. She said that she was going to call the sheriff. He begged forgiveness, promised to consult a psychiatrist, and she agreed to hold off contacting the police but said that he must never again treat her violently.

I was absolutely amazed that she had made that phone call.

## DISCUSSION

Domestic violence is a serious healthcare issue. Family violence is the leading cause of injuries to women and every physician needs to be alert to his patients' reports that she, or he, is in an abusive relationship.

What made this patient's report of battering so hard for me to deal with? First, I did not trust the patient's story. Each time she reported abuse I examined her carefully for signs of battering: bruises, tenderness, abrasions, and found nothing. Her previous psychiatric history also made me leery. Second, I did not trust the patient's behavior. She was very controlling (arranging her chair between me and the door, reading her list of illnesses instead of conversing) and her complaints about sexual deprivation, coupled with requests for hugs made me physically uncomfortable and more standoffish.

I'm not happy with the way I handled this patient. If she is really a victim of domestic violence, I would wish to be more emphatic about her need to seek help in a potentially lethal situation. And, after having put the matter to her so bluntly, I felt that I had joined her husband in the process of mistreating her. I was repaying her for the oppression I had felt at her hands and felt guilty about my behavior.

Nonetheless, to my surprise, my refusal to continue to play "Yes, But..." with her led to a change in her behavior. Perhaps it even led to a change in her husband's behavior.

What about my feeling of being oppressed? Surely I have to deal with the other features of that oppression. I must tell her that I would like her not to rearrange the furniture. I may have to accept her shorthand notes, but I could define my limitations in time and the number of problems that I can address in one visit.

# I WROTE IT DOWN!

Dr. Xylom: Hello, Henry, how have you been doing?

H: Not so good, Doctor. I still have that belly pain. I have to take Tums all the time.

X: My goodness! The acid blocker I gave you didn't work?

H: Oh, I didn't get that prescription filled. I forgot.

X: Forgot? Not too expensive then?

H: No, I'm on Compli-Care and they pay for prescriptions.

X: Well, what about elevating the bed head and not eating at night?

H: Oh yeah, I forgot those too. At my age it's sometimes hard to remember.

X: Really? You're only 52. Besides I wrote the suggestions down for you.

H: Yeah. Well I must have misplaced that note too.

X: What did you do? Anything I suggested? How about cutting down on the coffee and the beer?

H: Oh, I don't drink much beer, maybe a couple of six packs a week. And coffee, I guess that's about the same.

X: It all sounds about the same. Let's see. We did that X-ray study with the barium and it showed a lot of esophageal reflux. You have this pain in your upper abdomen and I think it is from irritation of the esophagus, esophagitis, right?

H: Yeah, I guess that's what you told me.

X: And we went through what you should do and I wrote it all down and it doesn't sound as if any of it took.

H: No, Doc, I guess I forgot.

## DISCUSSION

When patients pay to come hear our recommendations, why don't they follow our instructions?

This is really a question about adherence, what used to be called compliance. Studies have all shown that adherence statistics are much worse than we would like to believe. Patient adherence has to do with the patient's view of the seriousness of the problem, the simplicity and clarity of the therapy, and the patient's view of the doctor's interest and compassion. Above all, plans for actions that the patient must take must involve the patient in the planning. All such plans must include a collaborative involvement of doctor and patient.

This pair haven't yet reached such collaboration but the failure to date is a good reason for a discussion of the need for such collaboration.

X: Well, Henry, we aren't making super progress this way. Let's consider doing it differently. This pain is still bothering you?

H: Sure is.

X: And what are you able to do for it?

H: I dunno, Doc. I guess that's why I come to you.

X: OK, but I went over the things that I think will help. What of those are you able to do? Maybe it would help me to know better what problems arose in your remembering the medicines.

We might also consider the possibility that written instructions fail because the patient can't read. Or can't read our dreadful handwriting. If we have given him stock printed instructions from our file cabinet, we must be sure that these instructions really deal with his problems.

Perhaps we have to personalize them so that he understands they are specially for him, another sign that we care about him. We need to ask what we and the patient could do to avoid the difficulties. Ask what we can do to help. We may need to ask specifics: Can you read? Can you read my instructions? Where will you put the medicine? Will you see it there? Is there a better place? and so on.

All this may fall under the rubric of anticipatory problem-solving.

# I'M GOING TO BE ALL RIGHT,
# AREN'T I?

During this interview with Mrs. Phloem, her daughter sat silently by.

Dr. Xylom: Mrs. Phloem, I want to be sure that you understand what we've been saying. A lot of it can easily be confusing. Can you tell me how you understand what is wrong with you?

P: OK, Doctor, you told me that my gallbladder burst because it had cancer in it. And then some of the cancer had spread into my liver. You said that Dr. McClean wasn't able to remove all the cancer. But I feel pretty good now. I'm going to be all right, aren't I?

X: You surely are feeling better now. And I am glad that you have recovered nicely from the peritonitis when your gall bladder ruptured. But the cancer will probably cause trouble in the future.

P: Isn't there some sort of chemotherapy to cure it? Dr. McClean said you would take care of it.

X: I will surely stick with you, Mrs. Phloem. And I will do my best. But there isn't very good chemotherapy for this specific tumor and your rheumatoid arthritis may make it hard to use certain treatments.

P: Well, I'm sure that with you and Dr. McClean, I will be fine.

I'm going to be all right, aren't I?

X: Well, I hate to sound discouraging, but things probably won't be so fine. This sort of cancer spreads no matter what we do. It is unstoppable.

P: You mean I'm dying? Oh, I thought I was going to be OK. Dr. McClean said I would be OK. Are you sure? I felt better than for a long time. Now I feel just terrible.

## DISCUSSION

The doctor is distressed by his patient who is seriously ill and wants to be told an unrealistic good prognosis. The patient is unable to hear the bad news. What to do?

I think our job doesn't have to include beating the patients down and removing all vestiges of hope from their hearts. We can be honest and still leave hope, even denial, in place.

The doctor could say:

X: Well, of course we never know exactly what is in store for us. This sort of tumor can cause trouble in the future but we don't know how it is going to behave for sure. You may go a long time without trouble. In any case, you and I will work together and do the best we can as things go along.

Of course, this is also a good opportunity to talk about dying. There is a lot we need to know and now, while the patient is feeling pretty good, is a better time to think about the issues than later when she is sick.

X: Mrs. Phloem, I do want to know some of your feelings now, so I will have heard them if there ever is a time when you are quite ill and can't express your desires to me. I find that it helps me to know my patients' opinions of how they want to be treated, whether there is any specific treatment they don't want, especially if they are ever caught in a condition where they can't make their wishes clear to me. For example, if you ever have a stroke or are in a coma...

P: Oh, if that ever happens, I wouldn't want any extra things done.

What actually happened here? This patient eventually seemed satisfied with the discussion, but her daughter was not. The daughter took Mrs. P. to see the daughter's own gynecologist, who then referred her to an oncologist. The latter consultant, admitting that chemotherapy was useless, nonetheless placed her on a course of 5FU "because there was nothing else to do" and "because the daughter insisted." Mrs. Phloem never returned to Dr. Xylom and after a gradual decline of four months, was admitted to the city hospital with a fatal pneumonia.

So I view this interaction as a failure. I think the doctor was feeling hopeless and could have been more encouraging. And the patient's daughter, unheard in the dialogue, had strong concerns and ideas and eventually took over management. The critical flaw in this conversation was probably failure to hear the daughter.

# LIVING WILL

A: Dr. Platt, I brought in this living will. My friend gave it to me and I thought I'd want to tell you.

P: I see. And do you agree with all this??

A: Yes, I do. If I am ever hopelessly sick and can't tell you, I don't want any extraordinary things done to me.

P: I see. How about a few specifics. Say you have a stroke and after a week you still can't talk and can't eat. Would you like us to place a feeding tube in your stomach through the abdominal wall?

A: Well, what would happen if you didn't?

P: We could give you fluids for several days by vein and then for a few weeks by a tube down your nose into your stomach, but sooner or later we would have to decide to let you die of lack of food and water or to put a tube into your stomach through your belly wall.

A: Oh, I haven't thought of that. I'll have to think about it.

P: OK. How about a different problem. Suppose you get demented. That's what you call senility, what we call Alzheimer's disease. Suppose you are able to eat and drink but no longer make any sense, don't recognize people, and have to be kept at a nursing home.

A: That would be terrible.

P: Right. Then, suppose you get a pneumonia, an infection in the lungs. If we don't treat it, you will probably die. If we treat it with antibiotics you will survive, no better or worse than before. Would you want us to treat it with antibiotics?

A: Oh, I haven't thought about that.

## DISCUSSION

Lots of elderly people arrive in my office these days, bearing the paper work of a living will. They have a picture of massive technological intervention, not realizing that the more common dilemmas involve ordinary daily therapeutic decisions.

I find it helpful to give them common scenarios to consider. I make sure that one is the event of sudden unexpected death in hospital when they are admitted for other illnesses or operations.

Left without such guidelines, relatives are often uncertain and sometimes demand excessive medical efforts in hopeless situations. Our work is greatly simplified if we have had clear discussions with the patient ahead of time.[27]

Nance Cunningham, a medical ethicist at Yale, reminds me that we might also query our patients about their individual desires, not just what they don't want. For example, do you have a favorite sort of music you want played in your room? How awful to be mute and have to suffer from popular music or from the absence of music if you, like me, are a fan of classical music. Do you like pajamas or a hospital gown? Do you have a favorite stuffed toy? Is there anyone you want notified if you are unable to communicate and whom we might not otherwise look for? Would you like to be cared for in the hospital or at home or where? What else would you like us to provide for you if you become ill and unable to communicate?

# TOO SICK TO COME IN

Phone: Dr. Anneberg? This is Dr. Smooth. I'm glad I got ahold of you. I've been sick for three weeks.

A: My goodness! What sort of trouble are you having?

S: Oh, the same old thing. Short of breath and coughing. I've been too sick to come in.

A: I thought I saw you at that hospital banquet last week.

S: Yes, I thought I was a little better so I went to it.

A: And how are you treating yourself?

S: Well, you know I'm on the oxygen all the time. And I did start taking tetracycline two weeks ago. It might have helped a little, but now I'm back coughing up green sputum again. I thought you might pick something better than the tetracycline and call it in.

A: What decided you to call me just now, at 5PM?

S: Oh, you know, the nights are nasty. And I just realized that this had been going on for three weeks, time to get some help.

A: Are you taking your other medicines?

S: Yes, the diuretic and the bronchodilator just as before. And I use the inhaled steroids as you suggested, about five whiffs three times a day. That's when I think of it, of course. I miss a few of those mid-day doses.

## DISCUSSION

This physician patient, a retired radiologist with advanced obstructive lung disease, the result of a long smoking habit, presents several problems.

He may really be quite ill. Perhaps he needs emergency care.

Even if he's not so very ill, he's waited until it is quite inconvenient to see him in the office that day. And he wants telephone care.

What to do? Succumb to his request and order an antibiotic by phone? Very likely you can guess what antibiotic you will end up prescribing anyway. Invite him to come to the emergency room? Ask him to wait until tomorrow and come to your office? Does the fact that he is a doctor influence your choice?

I usually try to treat my physician patients just like my non-doctor patients. I tell them that.

Dr. A: John, I am not sure what the best thing is to do with you just now. But I usually try to treat my physician patients just like my non-doctor patients, not cutting corners or forgetting to do the work in a careful manner. I can see two reasonable choices. If you think you cannot make it through another night, I will meet you at the emergency room as soon as you can get there. If you think you can cope with one more night, I'd like you to come to my office tomorrow in the morning. Then I can examine you carefully, look at a sputum sample, and make a more sensible choice of therapy than I can do here over the phone. How does that sound?

S: You don't think just prescribing some ampicillin or some such would do the trick?

A: No, especially since the tetracycline didn't help. I really need to see your beautiful body and listen to your heart and lungs. It's hard to do that over the phone.

S: Can't I just put the phone to my chest and breathe deeply for you?

A: That's a great idea, but no, I think it wouldn't work. How about coming by at nine tomorrow morning? We will work you in.

S: OK, Lee, I'll be there.

# TERRIBLE SORE THROAT

A 26 year old woman came to an emergency room at 7PM with the following story. She had been ill for four days, suffering with a "terribly sore throat, fatigue, and fever. She felt "all in." There was no significant past history and she had been well until four days prior. The emergency physician examined her and noted large tonsils covered by purulent exudate. She had a fever of 101 degrees and the doctor thought she might have some splenomegaly. The upper cervical lymph nodes were large and tender. The doctor said that he thought she had a streptococcal throat infection but that mononucleosis was another possibility. He did a throat culture, a CBC, a Monospot test, and prescribed ampicillin four times a day for 10 days.

Two days later she returned again to the emergency department and said that she felt still worse. Her fever had not subsided, the throat was only marginally better, and she thought that her entire body was swelling up. The physician checked her throat culture from two days before and told her that she did have strep, that she would surely feel better in a day or two, and that she should continue with the ampicillin. He told her that nothing was wrong with her skin and that the sensation of "swelling up" was nothing to worry about.

Three days later she appeared in the office of another physician. She said that she thought she was dying and that she was worse and worse each day. The fever had reached 104 degrees, she was very weak and her skin was bright red and markedly edematous throughout. She was 20 pounds over her usual weight and the doctor surmised that it was all fluid. She appeared very toxic and was angry about what she considered to be cavalier treatment by the ER doctor who had "refused to hear my complaint of swelling" on her previous visit.

The physician called the hospital laboratory and found that the throat culture had grown group A beta-hemolytic streptococci but that the monospot test had also been positive. He knew of the association between mononucleosis and ampicillin-allergic reactions so he stopped her ampicillin, treated her with prednisone, and she made an uneventful recovery over the next week.

What should your strategy be when your patient is concerned about a physical finding that you cannot see on your exam?

## DISCUSSION

This patient was convinced that her ER physician had refused to hear her complaint. She thought that he treated her concern with disdain and that his arrogance led him to continue her antibiotic several days further, causing more suffering. She was mad enough to sue. When patients report that their doctor did not listen to them, they are very often right. There is no excuse for such behavior and neither patients nor our profession has to condone it.

However, frequently careful, considerate physicians may not be able to confirm physical findings noticed by the patient. The examination yields nothing. There is no satisfactory solution but to share your problem with the patient. "We have a real dilemma here. You note that your skin seems swollen, but I cannot identify it on my examination. You are probably sensing something that I can't pick up yet. I don't know what it means and may not be able to help until it gets worse, so that even I can see it." You can tell the patient that such situations are common, that they usually solve themselves by going away before the doctor can make a diagnosis, and that sometimes they get worse and then we can figure them out.

A discussion like this leaves the patient feeling that her opinion has been considered, that she has been heard, and that even if she is right, it is reasonable to go with your opinion for now.

# CAN I KEEP MY FINGER?

Dr. Strong: Good morning, Mr. Roberts. How are you feeling?

R: Well, OK, I guess. Except for my finger, of course. It still hurts a lot.

S: Let's take a look at it.

[He unwraps the dressing about the patient's left index finger, a finger that is clearly gangrenous, a dark purple distal to the metacarpal-phalangeal joint.]

R: It doesn't look good, does it, Doctor?

S: No, Bill, it doesn't. I think we better go ahead as we discussed.

R: Dr. Strong, I don't want to lose it. Please, I don't want to lose my finger. I want to keep my finger. Can I keep my finger?

S: You don't have to lose it. We'll give you a box to keep it in.

R: Oh, OK. (appearing reassured, according to the observations of the four other student physicians in the room at the time.)

What's going on here? Could a remark as outrageous as Dr. Strong's actually be reassuring? Should Dr. Strong's license to practice medicine be revoked? Is there any role for such outrageous comments?

## DISCUSSION

I heard this dialogue in 1963 when still a medical student. Dr. Strong, a hematologist at Stanford University, was conducting hospital rounds and had come upon a patient of his on the ward. I can't vouch for the word for word veracity of all of this dialogue, remembered at such a distance, but the critical lines burned themselves in my memory. At the time I was shocked by Dr. Strong's joking remark and could not understand why it seemed to be therapeutic to the patient.

Since then I have seen outrageous remarks used to good effect many times and have adopted the practice myself. The outrageous remark often is a sort of hyperbole, exaggerating the patient's symptom or his worry. For example, I have occasionally told a patient that the only test we have not yet done is an autopsy and that such a test would be a bit premature right now. To the surprise of any observer, such a remark seems to reassure my patient.

I believe that we must be careful with such outrageous and remarkable comments but that they can be used to lessen patient anxiety. To do so it is important that the doctor and patient already have a firm, comfortable, well-established relationship. The trust level already has to be quite high. And the doctor has to have done all his or her work, no examination half-done, no explanations left out. Then, if the doctor can joke a bit, I believe the patient may surmise that things can't be quite as bad as he imagined. The jest may then be therapeutic.

Is such a jest ever a failure? Sure. Nothing we do works all the time. But I can only remember one patient who gave me to know that his health was not a joking matter, that he expected total seriousness from me about anything having to do with his health. I apologized and refrained from jests from then on with him and we had a pleasant 10 year relationship together.

# YOU'RE NOT YOURSELF
# TODAY, DOCTOR

Dr. David says that he should have seen it coming. He was having a busy day when his office assistant told him that Ms. Credo had come in to be seen. Ms. Credo's visits often caused Dr. David to cringe. She was a retired nurse, full of theories of psychopathology about which she liked to lecture Dr. David. She liked to spend a great deal of time telling him about her right brain needs and her psychic features. On this visit, called in as a routine visit, Ms. Credo had told the office assistant that she was suffering with an erratic pulse and shortness of breath.

Fortunately, Dr. David had a medical resident working half a day in his office. Dr. Fawn went to see Ms. Credo and spent an hour reviewing her history and examining her. She emerged from the examination room to tell Dr. David that his patient was in florid heart failure and needed to be hospitalized, but lacked hospital insurance. To save time, before talking with Ms. Credo, Dr. David called the hospital and arranged for a special admission to a clinic service. He then went to see his patient.


D: I'm glad to see you, Ms. Credo. Dr. Fawn has told me what's been going on. We need to put you into the hospital to tune up your circulatory system.

C: Oh no, Doctor. I can't do that.

D: What do you mean, you can't? I just arranged for your admission. You have heart failure and need hospitalization.

C: Well, my biorhythms are too low to go into the hospital right now.

D: Never mind your biorhythms. You have to go in to the hospital. There's no other way about it.

C: Oh me. Dr. David, you usually don't talk that way to me. You don't seem to have any concern for my spiritual needs today. Is there something wrong with you? Is everything OK at home? You're not yourself today, Doctor.

D: Never mind what's going on with me and home. You're the patient, not me. You have to go right to the hospital. We can't do it any other way.

C: Well, if you think that, Doctor, I'm going home.

And, indeed she did go home. By the next day, Dr. D. was feeling a little guilty about his part in the fruitless interchange. He tried to phone her but, no answer. Finally, after a week of daily calls, she answered to tell him that she had spent the week in another hospital under care of another doctor, and now felt much better, thank you.

## DISCUSSION

What explains our sluggishness at recognizing that something is going wrong in the interview process? Are there several steps in that recognition? What gets in the way?

How should we recognize interview disasters in the making?

I'm not sure what the best sequence would be, nor that it would work for all of us. My own awareness of disintegration of the interview process seems to go in steps. First there is the 'Oh-shit phenomenon', simply an overwhelming awareness that something isn't working. This isn't the way I had planned my day. This isn't the way it is supposed to go.

Once aware that disaster has struck, I need to exert real force to stop whatever I am doing and just stand there. The important action is *stopping*. That's very hard to do. I can remember learning years ago that the most important safety maneuver for pilots is the 180 degree turn. And that is a very difficult maneuver to make. Not for the plane. It turns around with ease; but for the pilot, who has to make the decision. Once, flying directly towards a huge storm, I made that 180 degree turn. Once done, it was obvious and I knew it was right. Up to that instant it seemed far less obvious and hard to do. Similarly, in communicating with patients, your critical safety maneuver is to stop talking, stop questioning, simply stop whatever you are doing. You may have to tell your patient that.

Dr.: I need to stop for a moment. Something is going wrong and I need to think about it for a bit.

Once you have stopped, you can apply your thoughts to the new diagnostic puzzle, what is going wrong now? It helps to have a differential diagnostic  scheme for figuring out such puzzles, but even if you lack one, you will usually come to some reasonable hypotheses. Then you can ask your patient for help. Or you can ask for help before you come to any of your own hypotheses.

To repeat, the critical steps for dealing with interview disasters are:

1. Be aware that something is going wrong.

2. Stop engines

3. Ask what is going wrong now?

4. Enlist the patient in helping with that diagnostic puzzle and in remedying the problem

In this case, Dr. David had not interviewed or examined the patient. He had not yet attended to her psychosocial needs. When some things still need doing, we have to do them. This woman was not one to be bullied. She would cooperate when her cooperation was enlisted, but not until. And Dr. David was on a non-stop locomotive, no place from which to listen to his patient's concerns. It's no surprise that things went badly.

I am touched by the patient's inquiry about Dr. David's emotional state. Not a useful comment at that point, but still testimony of her concern for and trust of her physician. She could tell that he wasn't himself and let him know that she could imagine possible reasons. When Dr. David contacted her by phone a week later, she was glad to hear from him, eager to forgive him, and willing to come back to him in the future. It is amazing to me that our patients do tolerate and forgive us for a lot of obnoxious behavior. All we have to do is apologize and try to do better the next time.

# PULLING TEETH

Dr. Glitch: Hello, Mr. Peterman? I'm Dr. Glitch.

P: Peterson.

G: Can you tell me what sort of trouble you were having that got you into the hospital?

P: (slowly and softly) My foot. It, uh, it had a ...

G: You were having trouble with your foot?

P: Yuh. It was sore and they had tried to fix it and it wasn't, it didn't get better, it ...

G: Was it hurting? Did the foot hurt you?

P: Nope.

G: How long has the foot been hurting?

P: Doesn't hurt.

G: Which foot are we talking about, anyway?

P: This one. (wiggles left leg under bedclothes)

G: Which did you say? (He wasn't looking when the patient wiggled.)

P: Didn't say.

G: What other medical troubles do you have?

P: Don't have any. Except the prostate. And I itch.

G: Did you have a prostate operation?

P: Maybe, they did some operation.

G: So you came into the hospital because the foot hurt.

P: Didn't hurt.

G: How about other problems? Breathing? Pain anywhere else? Chest pain?

P: I dunno, I ...

G: Do you have diabetes?

P: I, uh, don't ...

G: High blood pressure? Taking any medicines?

P: No. Just the pills the doctor give me ...

G: OK. Any allergies?

P: Just the itching.

G: No medicines you're allergic to?

P: Uh uh.

G: OK, do you smoke?

P: Uh uh.

G: Well, let me take a look at your foot.


This physician had several things to say about the interview. First, prior to the interview he suggested that it was a waste of time to study aberrant interviews since he, in three years of medical residency training, had only had one interview that was problematic. Second, after the interview he allowed that this was a difficult one because the patient had contributed so little: "He was a tough patient." Finally he admitted that he asked a lot of questions but only because the patient was so hard to get any information from. "It was like pulling teeth," he said. And, he noted that this very large patient had a very little voice and sometimes he had difficulty hearing the patient.

What do you think about this sort of interview technique?


## DISCUSSION

This sort of dialogue is painful to watch. The four physicians watching this interaction noted that the doctor doing the interview missed many of the patient's comments, that the doctor used almost entirely closed questions, and that the patient became less and less communicative as the interview progressed.[28]

This sort of process is usually described as a "high control interview." Its characteristics are: the doctor talks a lot more than the patient; the doctor's main device is the closed question; the patient responds in shorter and shorter answers; and the doctor, sensing his unresponsiveness, presses harder and harder with tighter questions. In the end, the physician is usually dissatisfied. "It was impossible to get anything out of that fellow; he didn't want to talk to me." And the patient too is dissatisfied, often claiming, "The doctor didn't want to listen to me," and sometimes labeling the physician as arrogant. It is obvious in this interview that neither doctor nor patient heard the other very well, with misunderstandings thicker than ants at a picnic.

I have noted that this specific interview syndrome seems to increase in frequency as residents proceed through their medical residencies. That seems surprising and is worthy of comment. If we are teaching physicians how to be worse and worse, we ought to worry about the process. It seems that by the end of the residency, our residents think that the best way to take a history is to ask the key 250 questions. If so, no wonder they seem pressed to do so. And no wonder the patients are oppressed by them doing it.

This resident had amazed me by announcing that he had had only one communication mishap in his entire training program. He must be very good, I mused; I have mishaps every day. When, after this dialogue, he admitted that it had been a hard one, I commiserated with him. "The good news," I told him "is that you have now doubled your series of difficult interviews."

# I'M SORRY

The patient presented many complicated problems. She suffered from severe corticosteroid-dependent asthma, hypertension, diabetes, and now a new limb weakness that seemed unexplainable by any neurological or muscular disorder and that consultants had labeled 'hysterical' or 'conversion reaction.'

She was a heavy burden on the office staff and doctor, calling frequently, demanding more than her share of care, and probably was suffering from a chronic depression.

The doctor had had a long, hard day. Passing the examination room with Ms. Rose, he noted her chart in the door rack and cringed. Half way down the wall he remarked to his office assistant:

Dr. X: Do I have to see Susan Rose today? I don't think I can stand one more visit with her. She is such a crock.

Unfortunately, the patient was able to hear this disturbing remark and when the doctor came back up the hall and entered the examination room, she let him have it:

SR: (standing) You have no right to talk about me like that! I don't care what you think about me. You are like all those other doctors who blame me for my troubles and think they are better than human beings. You can take your doctoring and shove it. (crying) I don't care if you never want to see me again! I can find another doctor. That is the most hateful thing anyone has ever done to me.

What now?


## DISCUSSION

Have you never put your foot in your mouth? If not, don't be too confident that you will never do so. We are all capable of saying nasty things about other people, especially when we think we won't be overheard.

W.D. Ross, a Kantian ethicist, listed seven prima facie duties, ethical principles of behavior for human beings: nonmalfeasance (not doing harm), beneficence (doing good), justice, fidelity, gratitude, reparation, and self-actualization. It is reparation we need deal with here. When we do damage, we have to be prepared to apologize and try to make reparation. This is an opportunity, an obligatory need, for an apology. We must avoid the temptation to defend ourselves when we are caught out like this.

X: Susan, you are absolutely right. I don't know what led me to say what I said but it is altogether out of line. I am truly sorry. I can imagine that you are so angry that you will have to leave me. But I want you to know that you don't have to go, that I will still stick with you if you can stand me. I do apologize and I am contrite.

The doctor did apologize, the patient did elect to continue on with him, and their relationship seemed to improve dramatically from that moment on. This particular patient had never before been able to stand up to any person in authority about any matter. Doing it in so dramatic a fashion this time and finding that no lasting damage resulted, that they could continue on together, seemed to increase her trust and her self-confidence.

The doctor too benefited from the interaction. He was obliged to come to grips with his own fallibility and the potential for damage that he possessed. He was lucky enough to be able to respond out of humility and honesty, positions that are always best. He felt cleansed of a bad feeling and more like a doctor.

Amazing as it seems, this interaction that seemed so destructive led to a better doctor-patient relationship and an improved interaction thereafter.

# BIBLIOGRAPHY

## TEXTS ON INTERVIEWING

A. Browne, K. and Freeling, P. *The Doctor-Patient Relationship.* Churchill Livingstone, Edinburgh, 1976

B. Enelow. A.J. and Swisher, S.N. *Interviewing and Patient Care* 3rd Edit. Oxford University Press, NY, 1986

C. Cohen-Cole, S.A. *The Medical Interview: The Three-Function Approach.* Mosby Year Book, St. Louis, 1991

D. Coulehan, J.L. and Block, M.R. *The Medical Interview: A Primer for Students of the Art.* F.A. Davis, Phila. 1992

E. Balint, M. *The Doctor, His Patient, and the Illness.* Intl University Press, 1972

F. Lipkin, M. *The Care of Patients - Concepts and Tactics.* Oxford University Press, 1974.

G. Reiser, D.E. and A.K, Schroder, A.K. *Patient Interviewing - The Human Dimension.* Williams and Wilkins, Baltimore, 1980.

H. Bernstein, L., Bernstein, R.S. and Dana, R.H. *Interviewing: A Guide for Health Professionals,* 2nd Ed. Appleton-Century-Crofts, NY, 1974.

I. Levinson, D. *A Guide to the Clinical Interview.* W.B. Saunders Co., Phila., 1987.

J. Tumulty, P.A. *The Effective Clinician.* W.B. Saunders, Phila., 1973.

K. Mishler, E.G. *The Discourse of Medicine: Dialectics of Medical Interviews.* Ablex Publishing Co., Norwood, NJ, 1984.

L. Meichenbaum, D. and Turk, D.C. *Facilitating Treatment Adherence.* Plenum Press, NY, 1987.

M. Lipp, M.R. *Respectful Treatment.* Elsevier Press, NY, 1986.

N. Bird, B. *Talking with Patients,* 2nd Ed. Lippincott Co., Phila., 1973.

O. Kleinman, A. *The Illness Narratives: Suffering, Healing, and the Human Condition.* Basic Books, NY, 1988.

P. Mizrahi, T. *Getting Rid of Patients: Contradictions in the Socialization of Physicians.* Rutgers Press, 1986.

Q. Konner, M. *Becoming a Doctor - A Journal of Initiation in Medical School.* Viking Press, 1987.

R. Platt, F.W. and Mayer, D. *Case Studies in Emergency Medicine,* 2nd Ed. Little, Brown and Co., Boston, 1991

## ARTICLES OF INTEREST

1. Engel, G.L. The care of the patient: art or science. *Johns Hopkins Med J.,* 1977; 140: 222-232.

2. Korsch, B.M., Gozzi, E.K. and Francis, V. Gaps in doctor-patient communication. *Pediatrics,* 1968; 42: 855-871.

3. Bertakis, K.D., Roter, D. and Putnam, S.M., The relationship of physician medical interview style to patient satisfaction. *J Fam Practice,* 1991; 32: 175-181.

4. Fletcher, C. Listening and talking to patients. *Brit Med J.,* 1980; 281: 845-847, 931-933, 994-996, 1056-1058.

5. Platt, F.W. and McMath, J. Clinical hypocompetence: the interview. *Ann Int Med.*, 1979; 91: 898-902.

6. Quill, T.E. Recognizing and adjusting to barriers in doctor-patient communication. *Ann Int Med.*, 1989; 111: 51-57.

7. Smith, R.C. and Hoppe, R.B. The patient's story: integrating the patient- and physician-centered approaches to interviewing. *Ann Int Med.*, 1991; 115: 470-477.

8. Martin, A. Exploring patient beliefs: steps to enhancing physician-patient interaction. *Arch Int Med.*, 1983;143:1773-1775.

9. Suchman, A.L. and Mathews, D.A. What makes the patient-doctor relationship therapeutic? exploring the connexional dimensions of medical care. *Ann Int Med.*, 1988; 108: 125-130.

10. Bellet, P.S. and Maloney, M.J. The importance of empathy as an interviewing skill in medicine. *JAMA*, 1991; 266: 1831-1832.

11. Zinn, W.M. Transference phenomena in medical practice: being whom the patient needs. *Ann Int Med.*, 1990; 113: 293-298.

12. Jacobs, *et al.* Screening for organic mental syndromes. *Ann Int Med.*, 1977; 86: 40-46.

13. Brody, D.S. The patient's role in clinical decision-making. *Ann Int Med.*, 1980; 93: 718-722.

14. Brody, D.S. *et al.* The patient perception of involvement in medical care: relationship to illness attitudes and outcomes. *J Gen Int Med.*, 1989; 4: 506-511.

15. Quill, T.E. Partnerships in patient care, a contractual approach. *Ann Int Med.*, 1983; 98: 228-234.

16. Twain, M. The facts concerning the recent carnival of crime in Connecticut. In: *Great Short Works of Mark Twain*, 1967.

17. Williams, G.C. *et al.* The facts concerning the recent carnival of smoking in Connecticut and Elsewhere. *Ann Int Med.*, 1991; 115: 59-63.

18. Martin, A. and Coates, T.J. A clinician's guide to helping patients change behavior. *W J Med.*, 1987; 146: 751-753.

19. Benardo, M.A. and Mayerson, E.W. Patient-physician negotiation. *JAMA*, 1978; 239: 1413-1415

20. Barsky, A.J. Hidden reasons some patients visit doctors. *Ann Int Med.*, 1981; 94: 492-498.

21. Molde, S. and Baker, D. Exploring primary care visits. *Image: the J of Nursing Scholarship*, 1985; 17: 72-76.

22. Mann, P. *et al.* Depression among patients with a chief complaint of chronic fatigue. *J Affective Disorders*, 1989; 17: 165-172.

24. Hackett, T.P. and Cassem, N.H. Borderline Patients Groves, J.E. *Handbook of General Hospital Psychiatry*, 2nd Ed. PSG Publishing Co, Littleton, 1987.

25. Schlauch, R.W., Reich, P., and Kelly, M.J. Leaving the hospital against medical advice. *NEJM*, 1979; 300: 22-24.

26. Applebaum, P.S. and Roth, L.H. Patients who refuse treatment in medical hospitals. *JAMA*, 1983; 250: 1296-1301.

27. Gordon, G.H. and Tolle, S.W. Discussing life-sustaining treatment. *Arch Int Med.*, 1991; 151: 567-570.

28. Beckman, H.B. and Frankel, R.M. The effect of physician behavior on the collection of data. *Ann Int Med.*, 1984; 101: 692-696.

# ABOUT THE COVER PHOTOGRAPH

The cover was taken from an article about housecalls published in the *Rocky Mountain News* on April 29, 1983. The photographer, Laura Lynn Fistler, came along with me on a home visit to Nettie Pomarico, one of my favorite patients. The photo was provided by the Denver Public Library's Western History Department

Nettie died three years ago and I am no longer able to visit her, nor can I partake of the elegant repasts she used to provide following an invitation to "stay to take a cup of coffee." Nettie and I acquired each other when her prior doctor retired. At age 80, she wasn't eager to trust another physician, so she sent her daughter, Mary, to consult me first. Only after her daughter passed judgment and said that I was adequate did Nettie herself come. Then, since the relationships that were clearest in Nettie's mind were those of family, she dealt with me as another son. I worked on developing a doctor-patient relationship but this patient short-circuited the matter and invited me to join her family.

I think this picture has an unfortunate imbalance of height for a book about interview process. One would prefer both members at the same altitude. But Nettie had just told me of a touching problem, so I leaned over to touch her. And one could never achieve an overwhelming posture with Nettie anyway. She was a family matriarch who had been enormously effective in her community and her church. No one could miss her power and her control of her own destiny.

As with so many patients whom we care for and who then die, Nettie is often with me. Some days I wake with a start wondering why I haven't seen her lately. Then I remember. Some days I hear her voice reminding me that it was about time I came by to see her. Sometimes being a doctor is a lot like being a very old person—more and more of our friends are dead. Some days I think I am surrounded by dead folk as much as by live ones.

Thinking of Nettie, I remember her penchant for notoriety. I think she would have been pleased to be on this cover.

Thanks, Nettie.